T0197362

Taking Care of
Miss Bee Bee
STORIES BY A DAUGHTER EXTRAORDINAIRE

Cheryl Edwards-Cannon

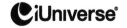

TAKING CARE OF MISS BEE BEE
STORIES BY A DAUGHTER EXTRAORDINAIRE

iUniverse books may be ordered through booksellers or by contacting:

iUniverse
1663 Liberty Drive
Bloomington, IN 47403
www.iuniverse.com
1-800-Authors (1-800-288-4677)

ISBN: 978-1-5320-2768-0 (sc)
ISBN: 978-1-5320-2769-7 (e)

Library of Congress Control Number: 2017910698

Print information available on the last page.

iUniverse rev. date: 09/13/2017

"Cheryl Edwards-Cannon speaks transparently from the heart about the joys and challenges of taking care of a loved one journeying through chronic illness. Get ready to laugh, cry, think, and above all else be encouraged!"

Shannon Cohen, Author of: *Tough Skin, Soft Heart: A Leadership Book* **about Growing Stronger, Better, and Wiser**

"Cheryl reassures us that God's grace is real. As a caregiver for her mother, she discovered a new depth of love and compassion. Her insight will become your blessings."

Dr. Cynthia McCurren, Dean of The Kirkhof College of Nursing, Grand Valley State University

FOREWORD

A friend of mine who had considerable knowledge of gerontology once told me that for many, if not most, people in this age, there are four stages to life:

1. The stage from birth to adulthood in which one grows and prepares for the duties and responsibilities of being an adult
2. The stage we might know as adulthood in which one is likely to find one's life partner, raise children, pursue a career, and prepare, at least financially, for retirement
3. The stage we know as retirement in which one hopes to have good health, sufficient resources to be free of the necessity of work, and time to pursue individual interests
4. The fourth and final stage, if one is lucky enough to live long enough, might be called decline

The decline stage might be abrupt or long. It is marked by physical and mental changes. In some it is marked primarily by physical aging. But in others, it may have much more to do with mental changes, from simple dementia to the full-blown disease we know as Alzheimer's disease.

Cheryl has done a marvelous job of describing that fourth stage through which her mother traveled. In her mother's case, the fourth stage was apparently quite long and ruthlessly defined by Alzheimer's disease. The perspective is that of the loving caregiver, Cheryl. The charm of the description lies in Cheryl's candor and humor.

Anyone with parents moving toward the fourth stage or who is personally approaching that state is likely to find this a useful and entertaining read. Enjoy.

Milt Rohwer, friend and former colleague

ACKNOWLEDGEMENTS

My thanks to Dani Phillips and LaRae Munk for their constant encouragement and confidence in me. You told me—for years—that my stories were worth telling. You were right. Love you, ladies!

◆

Also to my cheerleading team:
Lisa Edwards-Johnson, my sister;
Rosalyn Conway, my deep-thinking sister;
Willie Greene, my spiritual sister;
Renee Hayward, my play older sister;
and Shatara Morris, my adopted sister.

You ladies have been my confidantes, my sounding boards, and my encouragers. Thank you for making a space for me in your demanding lives.

◆

Any families motivated to write your own "Miss Bee Bee" stories, be encouraged. See the humor. Laughter will keep you sane.

SPECIAL ACKNOWLEDGMENT

Gentlemen, take a bow!

Many caregivers are women—mothers, sisters, sisters-in-law, and daughters. By their nature, women serve as caregivers more often than men. But there is a growing population of men who step into this role flawlessly. I have been fortunate to know eight of them:

- the Bloom brothers (Tim, Jim, Pete, and Mike)
- Robert Keith Browning
- John C. Smith
- Ralph Johnson
- Austin Reilly

You guys proved that men—yes, men—can be caregivers and be phenomenal at it. You provided remarkable care for your loved ones. You made me laugh, hugged me when words failed to provide comfort, and carried me when I could do no more.

Last, Larry C. Cannon, my husband, quietly took second place so I could keep my promise to Miss Bee Bee. Thank you.

INTRODUCTION

I have a reputation of being a good storyteller about my family, my assorted jobs, and those funny situations that make me wonder whether my life is one continuous comedy routine. I tell my informal audiences that I cannot possibly make this stuff up, that—trust me—this is what it is like to be me, Cheryl Edwards-Cannon. Personally, I feel that I am a much better storyteller than writer. My eighth-grade English teacher, Mrs. Schlabach, told me one day that I would be an author. If you are reading this, Mrs. Schlabach, wherever you are, perhaps you were correct, and I thank you for your confidence in me. Here I am on the umpteenth rewrite of my very first book. There is something about sharing my stories with others that brings laughter, which leads to great relief, not to mention that sharing is cheaper than seeing my therapist once a month. The story entitled "Ma'am, Please Step Out of the Car" was first printed in an edition of *Chicken Soup for the Soul: Alzheimer's and Other Dementias* (2014). Perhaps this book could have value after all.

Therefore, with encouragement from family and friends, I decided to write down stories about my mother's life with dementia. I wanted to share how the experience reshaped me into the person I am becoming. My journaling started in 2006 as a way of preserving the moments that brought me incredible joy that only comes from taking care of someone who eventually could not take care of herself. Most importantly, I wanted the stories to help others who are facing—or will face—the same challenges of taking care of loved ones. The most important thing I learned as her caregiver was this: meet her needs for where she is now and not for where I want her to be. Once I accepted the challenges of this disease, my life with her became easier to navigate.

Taking care of anyone who has a chronic and debilitating disease can be a devastating experience. It can erode relationships, drain financial resources, and leave families with a sense of hopelessness. Additionally, it may compromise the quality of the care the loved one needs. Frequently, families are not prepared or equipped to handle these challenges, which can quickly become an overwhelming and frightening experience.

Such was the case with my mother, Virginia, whom everyone called Miss Bee Bee. In 1998, at the age of seventy, Mom was diagnosed with dementia. I remember my dad and I met with her doctor, who, in a matter of minutes, confirmed her diagnosis, gave us a book on dementia, and ended the appointment. We left the doctor's office in silence, not fully understanding what we had heard, let alone what it meant. Although uncertain about what lay ahead, we were confident that we could work together and figure it out. But first we needed information to help guide our understanding of dementia and the plans we would need to make.

My sister and I started to research resources in the town where my parents lived to get as much information as possible, and we quickly learned that there was not much out there. Looking back on those early years, I realize that we truly did not have a clue about how difficult this journey would be for all of us. Initially, we thought it would be simple—Mom would remain at home with Dad looking after her, and this dementia thing would descend on her much later. I was just seventy-five miles away and could be home in just over an hour, and my sister, Lisa, who lived in Ohio, could help in other ways and would plan regular visits whenever possible. Easy, right?

We could not have been more wrong.

We had stressful moments while caring for Miss Bee Bee. She would inexplicably hide things, her driving was questionable, and getting her dressed was a daily challenge. Ultimately, we found laughter in absurd situations, found ways to keep her safe, and continued to love her unconditionally and hang on to our sanity. No matter how grueling things were, we never felt like we could not divide and conquer. When one of us needed a break, another would step in to provide the break.

Anyone who is a caregiver for an adult with dementia knows it is not unlike being a parent of a small child. Young children cannot take care of their own needs. Children need help in understanding the world around them. Children need protecting. There is a moral and humane obligation to provide care and oversight for society's most vulnerable: older adults and children.

Being a caregiver is not always an easy role to fulfill. Sacrifices are made, tough decisions decided, and numerous details organized. Nevertheless, I believe that with a fair amount of patience, planning, and support, it can be done effectively and be rewarding.

Therefore, I offer my stories with the utmost respect to everyone who is walking the path I walked. I hope that you can relate to my experiences and know that you are not alone. The demand for adult caregiving continues to grow as the population ages. Many will be summoned, as a result, to care for someone who can no longer care for him- or herself.

My family and I chose not to let Mom's diagnosis dictate our outlook on our lives or hers. We are a family of faith and believe that we will be successful no matter how difficult the challenges may be. We accept life's blessings graciously and humbly, and at the same time, we do not complain about the obstacles that block our way. In the end, we will find something to laugh about, be it at a funeral or family gathering. Humor will find its way to the situation. To those looking in from the outside, it may have appeared that I had everything figured out and tied up in a nice neat package to the point of appearing flawless, earning the title *daughter extraordinaire*. The truth is—there were times during Mom's illness that the load became complicated, heavy, and frightening. I was worried that I would make a mistake that would place both of my parents' lives in jeopardy.

The journey also taught me to take time for myself. I learned that it is all right for me to put myself first *occasionally*. I would schedule that spa day (my feet, hair, and hands will thank me), call my amazing girlfriends to catch up on all the latest gossip, or sit at home in absolute silence and just breathe. Most of all I learned that the load is a little easier to carry if I ask for help. I now know that I have family and friends who are always willing to come to my rescue.

In closing, I would like to say that this book simply embodies my reflections and thoughts about how this disease changed my life and allowed me to honor a woman who was loving, caring, and remarkable. I mean no disrespect and do not attempt to minimize the struggles, but I share my stories to celebrate the relationship I had with my mother, my hero, and my inspiration: Miss Bee Bee. If you are just embarking on your caregiver journey, I have listed several books and other resources that I found to be helpful at the end. Please read my stories with a smile, perhaps a tissue, and a feeling of hope and encouragement.

PS: Go ahead and laugh! It is okay. I do it all the time.

Cheryl Edwards-Cannon,
Daughter Extraordinaire

CONTENTS

THE CELEBRATION

Three months before my mother's planned retirement, I received a call from the president of the board of directors for the Benton Harbor Housing Commission, asking about the dinner celebration planned for her, which he and other board members would be attending. We both laughed about Mom's aversion to being in the spotlight, as she is very much a back-row individual. He asked if I thought I would have difficulty in getting her to attend, as there was a special surprise planned for her that evening.

I asked, "What kind of surprise?"

He told me that at the last commissioners' monthly meeting, the commission had decided in a unanimous vote to name this new building the Virginia Edwards Community Center. He went on to explain all the expanded services it would provide to the residents, as well as to the community. All of this directly spoke to the character Mom exemplified for her entire life. He said it was only fitting to name the facility in her honor.

I am quite certain the world stopped spinning for a few moments because I went numb as a huge wave of emotion came over me. Had I heard him correctly? A building named for my mother? This was a first for our family. This recognition was an unbelievable and extremely humbling honor. I am not exactly sure what I said in response to this news, but I know I was in tears and babbled out some sort of heartfelt thank-you and a promise that I would get her to the dinner even if I had to strap her to my back and carry her. The president asked me to keep this announcement a secret and that the commissioners would make the formal presentation at the dinner, when they would unveil the new sign for the building. The dinner was three months away—quite a long time to sit on this—but I said I would, and I did.

In the weeks that followed, Mom was constantly asking me if she would be required to say anything. "Cheryl, they won't make me say anything, will they? You know that I do not like doing things like that." In my head I was thinking, *Oh no, you won't have to talk because you will be speechless!* But to her, I explained that it would simply be a dinner, some people would say nice things about her career, and then we would all go home. That seemed to calm her until the next round of questions. Each time she asked about the dinner, I simply turned away with a little mischievous smirk on my face. Forgive me, Father, for I have fibbed to my mother.

For the next three months, I kept the secret as promised. I tried to limit my conversations with everyone so that nothing slipped. You know that adage "Loose lips sink ships." I got busy inviting our extended family from across the country, as well as family friends I knew would want to be there. Although a couple of times I came close to spilling the beans, I never tipped my hand. Mom and I went shopping for the ever-so-perfect dress and shoes for the evening. We made appointments to get our hair done, manicures, and makeup. I made sure she was going to be beautiful for her unveiling. As the big day approached, knots the size of Mount Rushmore were building in my stomach. I was certain I was going to pass right out and miss the whole event.

All the preparations were made, and the turnout was fantastic. More than 150 guests came to celebrate Mom's forty-plus years of service. The banquet room was decorated in gold, lavender, and white, which coincidentally matched the color of her new dress. Balloons and fresh flowers served as centerpieces on the tables draped in white tablecloths. Mom was presented with a perfectly matched wrist corsage, and my dad was given a coordinating boutonnière.

Soft dinner music filled the air that helped to transform the room into an elegant dining experience. The Housing Commission staff, all dressed in tuxedos, served as the wait staff and hosts for the dinner. People brought gifts and took pictures to commemorate the occasion. The executive director, Danethel Whitfield, emceed the program for the evening, which started after dinner. Danethel and I were high school classmates and over the last three months had exchanged many conversations about this event. When we walked into the room, she and I exchanged glances, signaling that everything exceeded our approval.

Mom's former employees recited their stories about her, most of which I had never heard before. They applauded her compassion, integrity, and commitment to people. The stories about their relationship with her moved me and others to tears. Each story revealed a deeper look into the remarkable person my mother was and the lasting impression she had on others.

A staffer who was a former tenant told a story that really drove this point home. She spoke of a challenging time in her life that led to an eviction from her apartment. It was my mother who had to serve the eviction notice. In usual Miss Bee Bee form, Mom delivered the notice with insurmountable respect and professionalism, encouraging her not to give up hope, but try to get things in her life straightened out and to reapply for housing. On moving day, Mom appeared at her apartment to help.

"C'mon, baby. The sheriff will be here soon, and you do not want him to put your stuff on the curb. Grab a box, and let's get things loaded," my mother said. Now, many years later, that evicted tenant was a model employee working alongside Mom.

The volume of comments made me realize just how much others valued and respected my mother. She was always phenomenal to me, but now I knew it was shaped by the people she served—always trying to make things a little better for anyone she met. These testimonies taught me that they loved my mother almost as much as I did.

Following a presentation by the city mayor and a representative from the US Department of Housing and Urban Development, it was time for the moment that had occupied my life for the last three months. The board president moved to the podium to make the last presentation for the evening. I could hardly contain myself. I sat at the head table with my parents, with Mom between my father and me. The podium was to our immediate left. He spoke about my mother as if he had known her for her entire life. His comments echoed the thoughts of many in attendance and prompted a few "amens" in agreement from members of the audience. Slowly the other commissioners joined him at the podium.

As he reached for the new building sign, which was discreetly lying on the floor behind him completely out of sight, I heard him say, "We've known Mrs. Edwards for a long time. I even went to high school with her daughter Cheryl. This center will provide resources so that people can research and apply for jobs in the new computer lab. There's a small but safe playground where children can play. The banquet room, where we are now, can be used for all kinds of gatherings and events. All of these characteristics are demonstrated by Mrs. Edwards. Therefore, in a unanimous vote by the Benton Harbor Township Commissioners, it is only fitting and proper that this building be named the Virginia Edwards Community Center."

I turned to look at Mom as the room erupted into a thunderous applause and a standing ovation. She broke into tears and quickly covered her face and bowed her head. Guests rushed to the head table to hug and congratulate her. I put my arm around her shoulder to support her, but I had just as much difficulty controlling my own emotions.

My dad, on the other hand, was in complete disbelief and kept repeating, "What? What? What? They named a building after you? What? What?"

You see, my dad was a celebrated police officer and was often featured in the newspaper for something or other. However, tonight it was all about celebrating Miss Bee Bee. He soon regained his composure and joined in congratulating her along with everyone else. He had always appreciated and respected her for working behind the scenes. But it never crossed his mind that his wife would ever be held in such high regard. It was a comical moment, to say the least.

After a few emotional minutes, Mom collected herself and decided that she did want to say a few words after all. She strutted confidently to the podium with the attitude, "I have got something to say." She was eloquent, reflective, and grateful for the honor. She thanked her husband for being supportive of her career but then she looked at me while saying, "I have a daughter who was keeping secrets from me, and I will deal with her later."

Mom shared several of her own stories about her life and career with the Housing Commission, the staff, who had become like her children, and all the tenants she met and looked after. She spoke of the importance of family and having a strong work ethic and the value of a good education that would enable anyone who wanted to pursue a successful career to do so. Standing just four foot nine behind that podium, she glowed and made me so proud of her that I wanted to continue her legacy, knowing that I had some big shoes to fill.

Today the Virginia Edwards Community Center provides services and resources for families and the community. The blight that once existed in the nearby neighborhoods has since been replaced with new homes, manicured lawns, and a state-of-the-art Boys and Girls Club.

For the daughter of a laborer and a domestic worker from Princeton, West Virginia, this was the most memorable event of her life. We did not realize it then, but this chapter of her life was closing to make way for another life-altering experience for all of us.

A LIFETIME OF CARING

My mom, Virginia Browning Edwards, held many titles to a wide variety of people: wife, mother, daughter, sister, aunt, and best friend. Mom was the fourth of five children born to William and Edna Browning of Princeton, West Virginia. My grandparents married on August 16, 1920, and remained married until William's death in 1948. William worked as a custodian, as many did in the early 1900s. The hours were long, and the work was brutal. Despite the meager wages, he provided a home for his wife and five children, while Edna made a living as a domestic. A very strong, confident, and proud woman, Edna continued to provide for her family following her husband's death. The oldest son, Frank, built a business as a licensed electrician, Sue was a lifelong educator and community volunteer, and Bob made his living as a laborer but always aspired to turn one of his many invention ideas into a financial coup. Sam, the youngest child—and often Mom's partner in crime—made a career out of serving in the US Navy.

Neither William nor Edna had a formal education beyond high school, but together they built a home on Craig Street in Princeton, West Virginia, and lived there for more than twenty years. Their home was well maintained, and I suppose for the time and location, it would have been considered a fancy house. It had running water, an attached water closet (bathroom to those unfamiliar with the term), three bedrooms, and a parlor. I remember the magnificent trees on their property, which seemed to go on forever, or so it appeared to a ten-year-old girl. The house had a long porch with a swing that would creak when swung back and forth. I only have memories of the house on Craig Street; it was destroyed by fire in 1968.

It was the tradition of the time that a family would continue to live under one roof until you either married and purchased a home of your own, left for college, or joined the armed services. The Browning family was no different. They were an honest, hardworking, well-respected family in this small southern community where everybody knew everyone else. Everyone attended the same church and shared in the economic struggles of that era.

Mom's brother Sam introduced her to future husband, Alfred, in 1946. Tall, lean, and handsome, with wavy black hair, Alfred was always impeccably dressed and always had a few dollars in his pocket. He immediately caught Mom's eye and captured her heart. He also had four siblings, who eventually moved to Princeton to a house just a stone's throw away from the home on Craig Street. At the time, Alfred worked in the coal mines in southwestern West Virginia, but he also had career aspirations for his life. After a brief courtship, they married on September 28, 1949.

Now all the other siblings on both sides were married and out of their parents' houses. But in the 1940s, job opportunities for men were limited to the coal mines or farms, and employment as a domestic was the only option for women. In search of better lives, both families, the Brownings and the Edwards, packed up and headed north to a little town called Benton Harbor located in southwest Michigan near the shores of Lake Michigan. In fact, my dad's brothers and sisters remained in Princeton and eventually moved into Mom's childhood home on Craig Street.

Each family purchased a house within walking distance of the other. I am certain that there was many a long conversation during the migration north as to, "Who will Edna live with?" In the end, my grandmother, at Mom's request and Dad's consternation, lived with us for about eleven years. Shortly after the birth of my sister, Lisa, in 1962, my grandmother moved to a duplex that was next door to her oldest son Frank's home. Edna was just a five-minute walk from her daughter Sue's home, as well as my parents' home. In total, the family from West Virginia lived near each other for more than sixteen years.

My parents had three children born five years apart, the reason being to have only one child in diapers at a time. That was Mom's rule. I am the oldest, followed by my brother, Chad, and then Lisa, the youngest. Not only were we born five years apart, but we were also born on Monday, Tuesday, and Wednesday, morning, afternoon, and evening. We grew up in a home where integrity and honesty where expected. We were surrounded by daily examples of family values, social responsibility, and respect for all. Although our career paths are quite different and we live far apart from each other, we still reflect the training from our childhood instilled in us by our parents, grandparents, aunts, and uncles.

Mom's given name was Virginia, which gradually evolved to Miss Bee Bee (probably because she could not pronounce the letter V). She was a born caregiver before there was a name for it. She simply took care of people. Early in her life, she was the caregiver for her father, William, who became gravely ill and had to be cared for at home until his death in 1948. Thirty-five years later, she was called to do the same for her mother.

My grandmother aged gracefully into her nineties and became the matriarch of the family. For most of her life, Edna lived independently and was quite capable of making her own decisions. But when the time came, Mom provided companionship and support and addressed all of Edna's needs to make her comfortable and keep her safe. The relationship between my mother and my grandmother was respectful and quite sincere. They loved each other and maintained unwavering trust in each other. Bee Bee seemed to smooth out my grandmother's rough edges and brought out a kindness in her.

Nevertheless, it has to be said that Edna was selective about who she liked and very selective about who she did not like—and that included her fourteen grandchildren. She was not particularly crazy about half of us, and we embarrassingly felt the same about her. Edna was not a warm and loving grandmother you wanted to cozy up to for milk and cookies. Instead, she was a firm and forceful woman, not to be questioned or argued with. Those who felt courageous enough to challenge her authority rarely had a second opportunity to do so. She was a devoted Christian who attended church regularly, paid her tithes, and prayed three times a day. Her behavior, however, showed us a different side. My mother liked Edna, so I made the attempt to do the same.

Edna was an only child and endured a difficult childhood. My grandmother spoke very little about her childhood, leaving us to believe it was a painful time in her life. She was reared for the most part by her stepmother. After her father remarried, he invited Edna to come live with him and his new wife. Her biological mother also remarried and had three more children from that union. Edna's recollections reminded me of the fairy tale of Cinderella, where my grandmother was responsible for the housekeeping and chores while her stepbrothers and stepsisters were allowed to do other more enjoyable activities. Edna's sadness about her childhood piqued my curiosity, and it made me want to know more. Her face said it all. I never pressed the point to probe further.

At the tender age of eighteen, my grandmother married William Browning and started a new life that brought her freedom and a chance to live. Now she could have a family of her own with a husband who loved her unconditionally. Edna could finally put her painful secrets away as best she could and start a life that had purpose and meaning.

One year we had the opportunity to host a family reunion at Edna's birthplace in Wytheville, Virginia. We held a church service on the land where her childhood home stood. It was there my grandmother spoke about her life growing up in the south during pre–World War I. I remember her appearing to be so strong and full of purpose and conviction. Her childhood life may have scarred her, but to her great credit, she was a survivor who outlived most of her family.

Edna continued her career as a domestic after the family moved to Michigan. She worked for a family in the neighboring town of St. Joseph. She worked several days of the week, cooking, cleaning, and attending to the needs of that family. My grandmother owned a car but never learned how to drive. Therefore, someone from the family would have to take her to work and remember to pick her up at the end of the day. I remember my grandmother wearing a perfectly pressed gray and white cotton uniform to work. Her apron was tied neatly behind her, and a nearly invisible hair net was on her head.

One summer when I was about twelve years old, my mother asked me to go to work with Edna to help her with a dinner party that this family was having. Not having a clue of what I was in for, I agreed because my mother asked me to help out. Little did I know what was in store for me. We entered the house through a side door that led directly to the kitchen. Immediately, my grandmother set to work to get organized before the guests arrived. I am still not sure how I got drafted for this tour of duty because cooking has never been my true calling, but Mom asked me to help and I could not say no. So, there I was in this lady's kitchen pretending to know what to do with her food. Very dangerous situation.

After helping Edna to get dishes and other serving pieces set out, I wandered from the kitchen into the living room, drawn by the family's piano. I was in my seventh year of piano lessons and wanted to play it. Edna was horrified when she heard me playing a few notes. She moved swiftly and abruptly to remove me from the room. She made it very clear that I was not to leave the kitchen and dared me not to go anywhere else. The lady of the house appeared just moments later to give Edna further instructions for the evening. All I could hear was my grandmother's barely audible response of "Yes, ma'am" or "No, ma'am." I thought, *Who does this lady think she is, to talk to* my *grandmother that way? Who is this woman to reduce this powerful grandmother of mine to a small, childlike figure?* I could not reconcile this moment with my grandmother's stubbornness and domineering personality. Then I thought, *Could it be that this woman has the power to take Edna down a peg or two? I must tell the other cousins!*

I knew then that I would never come back to that house or do the kind of work my grandmother had done for most of her adult life. This experience taught me two things: I did not want to do that kind of work. To wait on people who could perfectly come and get their own parsley-laced sandwiches? Work that demanded that I be submissive and condescended to? No way. No how. Not in this lifetime or the next. Second, it confirmed that I was college bound right after high school. Period. College would prepare me for a meaningful career and endless opportunities. All I had to do next was finish the next six years of middle and high school and I would be on my way.

The scene between the lady and my grandmother was uncomfortable and confusing. Why did my grandmother act in such a meek way? Why did I have boundaries that prevented me from exploring places filled with lots of interesting objects that mesmerized my imagination and enticed me to take a closer look? In retrospect, it really spoke of the life she had experienced since coming into this world—a life that was foreign to me at the time. Perhaps my parents used this as a teaching tool to ensure that I kept focus on my education and making wise decisions for my life. They were probably right.

My grandmother and I had our contentious moments off and on throughout our lives, but over time, we grew closer and found ways to get along. I appreciated her tenacity and strength. She in turn became less critical of me and softened her tone when we talked. I tried to see the good in my grandmother, and I would like to think she saw the good in me.

Edna finally retired at seventy years old and enjoyed life by going to church and traveling with friends and family. She hung up her uniform and apron and devoted herself to only cooking for her family every holiday. She continued to live independently for the next nine years. As her grandchildren started to grow up, we took turns transporting her from place to place. We confidently drove her around town to take care of her personal errands or to visit friends.

My grandmother fell and broke her ankle when she was seventy-nine years old. The break never healed correctly, resulting in her walking with a noticeable limp. It became more difficult for her to get around, but she managed. A couple of years later she fell again and fractured a hip. Although she healed well from that experience, she never walked again, more out of fear rather than physically not being able to. For the rest of her life, my grandmother used a wheelchair to get around.

As Edna became convalescent, Mom, while working full-time outside of the home, became her caregiver. We moved her to a house closer to my parents to make it easier for Mom to watch out for her. During this time, I watched and learned from my mother how to manage and balance a full work schedule, accommodate the needs of her mother, and care for her own family. As time moved on, my grandmother increasingly depended on my mother for everything: meals, laundry, companionship, and a sense of security. Frequently, I would spend the weekends at home helping and giving Mom a much-needed break. I had learned how to be her when she and my dad needed to get away and spend time doing things they enjoyed. I learned how to anticipate what Edna needed and to keep myself organized to ensure consistency with Mom's routine.

By this time in our lives, we had lost my uncles Frank and Sam just two weeks apart. Aunt Sue had relocated to Dunnellon, Florida. Uncle Bob lived next door to where we moved Edna, but the caregiver role was not his calling. This left Mom to be the giver of care for more than ten years. She never complained about her exhaustion or the strain it placed on her marriage. She merely did what she had to do to take care of her mother. Eventually, Mom hired some in-home health aides to provide the around-the-clock care for Edna, which allowed Mom to catch up on other events happening in her life.

Edna lived to be a very seasoned ninety-two years old and died peacefully on July 25, 1994. She had suffered a stroke and never regained consciousness. I sat with her for hours hoping she would respond to my voice and talk to me. That was not to be. Just twenty-four hours after I left her side, she slipped away for good. Mom was with her at the end and described what that experience was like. She was sitting near the window reading her Bible when a bright light lit the room, and a strange, serene silence covered the sound of the machines and Edna's breathing. Then she felt a calm presence as Edna's breathing stopped quietly and gently. Not needing a confirmation of death, Mom knew that her mother had made the transition from life on earth. Edna's passing meant that her life as the matriarch of our family was now over.

My mother asked me to plan the funeral service for Edna, and as expected, I agreed. I thoughtfully wrote the obituary to honor her memory and the legacy she left behind. She outlived two of her children and was the grandmother not only to the fourteen of us but also to eleven great-grandchildren. I invited all the grandchildren to sing "Rock of Ages" at the service since it was Edna's favorite hymn, under the direction of my sister, Lisa, and me on the piano. Edna would have been satisfied and proud. Despite how we all felt about her, we were able to set aside our feelings and celebrate the woman that was: Edna Leona Richardson Browning.

Remember—I said that my family will find something funny at any family gathering, and Edna's funeral was no different. Nearly twenty years after her passing, my cousin Renee was voted to tell me that the only reason they agreed to sing at the funeral was their love for Miss Bee Bee and me. Since Renee was the oldest cousin out of the fourteen of us, she was drafted. She said that it had nothing to do with a deep-seated love for our grandmother. Our performance at Edna's funeral somehow gave them confirmation that she was actually dead, never to terrorize any of us again. With that declaration, I was left speechless for a few minutes, but later Renee and I laughed until we could hardly breathe. I wondered why none of my cousins cried for our grandmother. Now I know why.

As this chapter was closing, another was beginning.

LIFE MOVES ONWARD

Edna's passing allowed Mom to get back to work and focus on her career and herself. She and Dad started to make plans to travel and enjoy this season of their lives. They were reconnecting with friends and family. It was a wonderful time in their lives following the ten-year stint spent providing care for Edna. Things appeared to be back to normal in the Edwards house.

My mother enjoyed a long career with the Benton Harbor (Michigan) Housing Commission. She started out as a bookkeeper and was promoted to manager, then finally assistant director of the Benton Harbor/Benton Township Housing Commission. During her lifelong career, her favorite assignment was managing the Harbor Towers Senior Center, a five-story apartment building located near downtown Benton Harbor, which about one hundred tenants called home. She affectionately referred to these tenants as her babies. She checked on them daily to make sure that all of their needs were taken care of, and she would always find the time to listen to their stories from their childhood. They had grown accustomed to seeing her regularly, and she never disappointed them. At the end of her workday, after arriving home, Mom would share a humorous story about Mr. So and So or Miss So and So. It was apparent that both tenant and landlord shared mutual feelings toward each other, making her visits worthwhile.

During her weekly visits, Mom would occasionally find a tenant who had died during the night, and she would see to it that their funeral arrangements were handled efficiently and with Mom's signature compassion. She felt a moral obligation to attending to a resident's final arrangements out of the respect she had for each of them. It was an essential ingredient of her character to simply care about people. For some, Mom was the only family they had, and they looked forward to her weekly visits. Many residents grew to see her more as their daughter and not as their landlord. These relationships taught me early lessons of what it meant to be a caregiver, to be in service to others. However, I had no idea the impact these lessons would make on my life.

Mom accepted the position of assistant executive director of the Benton Harbor/Benton Township Commission. The move required her to pack up, say goodbye to her babies, and move across town to another office about five miles away. For the next four years, she enjoyed the challenges of the new job, as well as connecting with new residents moving into the area and hiring young and energetic staff members.

Just a few months into her new assignment as the assistant director, Mom fell down on the back porch on her way to work and broke her ankle. She required surgery and was in a cast for several months. It is unclear what caused the fall; she said that she did not trip or stumble, but instead her bones simply gave way and down she went. Fortunately, my dad was at home at the time and was able to get her to the hospital. He called to tell me what had happened, and of course, I rushed home to be with her. Mom was not surprised when I walked into her room, as she knew that "her oldest would be showing up at any moment."

Like my grandmother, Mom had a history of falling and breaking bones. As a newlywed, she was playing softball one afternoon, hit an amazing ball to center field, and made a mad dash to first base, where a tree trunk served as the first base marker. She fell over it, breaking her leg. Another time, she tried to catch a heavy glass ashtray with her foot and broke her foot in several places.

Fortunately, Mom healed completely from her most recent mishap and seemed to get back into her routine in record time. She did not use a wheelchair, walker, or cane. She figured out ways to get herself around the house and at work based on sheer will and determination. I believe Mom's energy and high level of being active allowed her body to heal quickly. She did not require any follow-up surgeries, and after a few sessions with a physical therapist, she was as good as new.

One thing was different this time, however. Every so often Mom would comment to me, "I fell so hard that my head shook." As she said this, she kept touching the side of her head. I thought, *What an odd comment to make.*

After some time, perhaps several months after the fall, I noticed that her behavior had become a bit different, but for the most part, I dismissed it. The significance of her comment about the fall would eventually make sense but not for nearly a year.

Throughout the next year, a few times caused me to pause and ponder some of the events that occurred at my parents' home—like the time I found a cup of laundry detergent in the refrigerator or a peanut butter sandwich—partially eaten—in the nightstand drawer. She would have sudden moments of extreme anger and just as quickly, would calm down and not recall the outburst that occurred just seconds prior.

At the time, the most unsettling incident was the time Mom left the house to go to an appointment a few miles away. She arrived just fine, but during her drive back, some close friends about ten miles north of her home spotted her. Luckily, they thought it was odd for her to be out that way and alone. Somehow, they were able to get her to pull over to find out what was going on. It turned out that she was uncertain about her whereabouts but tried to play it off in a joking manner. Not willing to risk her driving herself, one of the friends got into her car and drove her back home.

Another troublesome incident happened when Mom traveled with a group to Saint Louis, Missouri, for a weekend-long conference.

The group rode the shuttle to the Saint Louis airport for the trip back; others left the group and rented cars to drive to various destinations around the country. While my dad and I are clear how she got to the Saint Louis airport, we do not know why Mom did not board the plane when it was time. For hours, Mom remained alone at the Saint Louis airport, apparently unable to ask for help or to even sort out the events of the day.

The closest airport to Benton Harbor was in South Bend, Indiana, about thirty-five miles to the south. We were expecting Mom to fly there, where Dad would pick her up. We were alarmed when she did not arrive back in Benton Harbor as scheduled with her other friends. Dad waited at the South Bend airport, hoping that she would be on the next flight. Finally, he drove back home in hopes of finding her there; perhaps someone else offered a ride home.

Unaware of any of this, I called home that evening to hear how the conference went. Dad answered, and instantly, I could hear the stress and anxious alarm in his voice as he related the day's events. He asked if she had called me. I told him no as I felt myself tensing up. We both called the airlines, the airport, and her friends to try to locate her. No one had spoken to her since the group said their goodbyes in Saint Louis. Where could she be?

Finally, at about three in the morning, she finally called home to tell Dad that she was at the South Bend airport and to come pick her up. It was clear that she was agitated, upset, and tired. We were relieved that she was safe, unharmed, and back at home. Dad and I decided to wait until another time to ask her about what happened. However, the only thing I was able to wrestle out of her was that she did, in fact, call home but did not leave a message on the answering machine. The phone would ring and ring as Daddy slowly navigated his way to answer it. However, as soon as the answering machine picked up, Mom hung up. (You have to remember these were the days before voice mail and caller ID.)

After experiencing these and other changes in Mom's behavior for about a year, Dad had her checked out by their family doctor.

The diagnosis confirmed what we all reluctantly suspected: she had early onset dementia, her condition would worsen over time, and there was no cure. Eventually, simple tasks such as eating and dressing would require assistance. As the disease progressed, she would eventually decline to a state of total dependent care. Worse yet, we were told that the lifespan of someone with this disease varies from a few short months to about ten years. Although some medications could help to slow the progression, nothing could reverse or cure it. The doctor wrote a prescription for a drug to help slow the process of memory loss—but it would only be effective for perhaps a year or two.

Now the pieces of this puzzle were starting to fit, and the picture was disheartening and scary. A thousand thoughts ran through my mind. *Is dementia painful? How can I help her? Help Dad? Help them?* I had a million questions and needed answers—fast!

I come from a family that faces challenges head on. We pulled together to make this journey as painless, loving, and meaningful as we could—for all of us. We never felt sorry for ourselves that this was happening to Mom; instead, we believed that God would provide the tools and strength needed to get us through this.

I know what you are thinking: turn to Google! Let me put this in perspective. Google didn't come into existence until 1998, the same year Mom was diagnosed. Back then, resources were scarce, if they existed at all. I contacted anyone I could find to help me understand better what we would be facing and what we should be doing. I met with doctors, attorneys, financial advisers, and our insurance agents. Dad joined a support group for caregivers to help him cope with the new role he would be playing. I went headfirst into learning what I could about dementia and Alzheimer's disease.

Mom continued to work as assistant executive director of the Benton Township Housing Commission and accomplished a great deal for nearly two years. By then, it was becoming apparent that the disease was progressing, and it was time for her to retire fully. She and Dad made that decision together and announced it to her staff, who could sense that something was different with her as they accepted her decision to leave the organization where she had spent forty years of her life.

It was at this point my life changed in a most remarkable way. The years that my parents poured into me the sense of responsibility and knowledge came full circle; insisting that I learn this and that about legal, financial, and medical affairs now served a purpose. I knew that it would be up to me to take a leadership position in our family to navigate the most significant event of our lives. The acceptance did not come without fear and uncertainty, but those feelings were suppressed with the confidence that they taught me well. I was prepared.

Let me share my stories.

A MOTHER'S ENCOURAGEMENT

For seven years, I worked for a commercial furniture manufacturer located in Grand Rapids. Grand Rapids is known as "furniture city" thanks to the large concentration of first residential, then office furniture companies in the area. The company I worked for was the second-largest manufacturer in the industry, where I had a very good career and received several promotions. It was a great place to work, where I found many long-lasting friendships in its close-knit, family-like atmosphere, and multiple generations enjoyed long, productive careers.

It was during the summer of 1995, three years before Mom's diagnosis, that tragedy struck my workplace when a young man I'll call Keith, out of respect for his family, a summer student employee, was killed in a hi-lo accident while working in one of the manufacturing plants. Just twenty-two years old, Keith was studying at a local college to become a paramedic. Well-liked and personable, Keith took a great deal of pride in his work, and his death sent shock waves throughout the company. To compound the tragedy, Keith's parents were also employed by the company and were at work when the accident happened.

As word of the accident spread, an eerie quietness permeated both the office and the plant. Some people wandered aimlessly in disbelief, while others grieved openly. The whole experience seemed surreal, unbelievable. There were no words that could explain why such a young life was lost all too soon. The accident sent our loving, family-friendly community into an emotional frenzy unlike anything in the company's hundred-year history.

A few days later, funeral arrangements were finalized, and so many friends, families, and employees planned to attend that a larger venue was needed to accommodate everyone.

John, a coworker of Keith's father, was asked to sing "The Lord's Prayer" and "The Old Rugged Cross" at the funeral, and I agreed to accompany him on the piano. I had studied classical piano for thirteen years and had played at many parties, weddings, and other celebrations, and John and I had performed together at a number of church events. However, I am personally not comfortable at funerals, let alone playing at one, and I expressed my apprehension. But we were both committed to delivering a performance that would give some small comfort and peace to the family.

John and I rehearsed two days before the service, and it was disastrous. Neither one of us could get in sync with the other. I kept making mistakes; John kept losing the key or would forget the words. It just was not coming together the way it needed to—the way we wanted it to. In frustration, we cut rehearsal short and agreed to try the next day—but we were running out of time. The funeral was set for the following morning.

I needed some words of encouragement and consolation from someone who knew the right words that would help me to get it together. So naturally, I called Mom. She would know what to say to me to calm my nervousness, anxiety, and uncertainties. A gentle, kind nurturer who possessed the power to make you feel great when you are down or doubtful, she was my go-to person, my cheerleader, and my champion. Many times, she helped me navigate the challenges I had faced throughout my life. Every time, Mom came through with the right words to move me through my fears—until this time.

I called Mom to tell her about the disastrous rehearsal and how afraid I was. Afraid that I would hit the wrong notes. Afraid that I would be consumed by grief and simply unable to play. I stopped talking, and the line went silent as I waited anxiously for a response.

My mother spoke slowly and firmly. She said, "Cheryl, this isn't about you. So stop it. You get your fear and anxiety behind you and put the face of God in front of you. This family has lost their child. You go and play for them so that they can be in peace. Let God use your talent to give this family comfort, as much that can be given at this time. Do not make it about you and your fear. You know what to do. Now go and do it."

I was speechless and could feel myself tearing up. She had never spoken to me this way. I needed encouragement and a phone hug, and she brought me up short with a reality check. I mumbled a few words of appreciation and told her I would talk to her later. Then I hung up the phone.

On the day of the funeral, there was a horrendous thunderstorm during my drive into work. As I navigated the heavy downpour, I prayed for God to take my hands and help them find the right keys to deliver a perfect performance for this family. I acknowledged to God that he was in control and asked for him to send me strength to do what I'd been asked to do. If he wanted me there, he would take control of the weather, as well as my car, to ensure a safe arrival.

John and I arrived at the church early so we could settle in and I could warm up for a few minutes. We sat in the choir loft in full view of the hundreds of people arriving to pay their respects. Some guests waved from their seats, surprised to see us sitting there. The company's CEO and chairman of the board sat near each other and nodded to us.

The officiating pastor signaled for us to begin. We began with "The Lord's Prayer," and John's voice filled the sanctuary. It was a magnificent performance. We felt each other's emotion and passion. Without a doubt, God was with us; it was the best performance we had ever done.

As the last note faded, I looked up from the keyboard at Keith's mom, seated in the front row. She smiled and nodded her head at me. At that moment, I knew we provided what she needed at that time. I had delivered my best to her and her family. I fought to hold my tears back and returned a loving smile back to her.

The service continued with a thoughtful and inspiring eulogy by the pastor and concluded with our rendition of "The Old Rugged Cross." To say that everyone was visibly moved would be an understatement.

I don't have much actual recollection of playing that day. However, whenever I listen to a recording of the service and hear me playing that magnificent baby grand piano, I know in my heart that I played my absolute best for this family. I do not think I have ever played that well since. My mother was right. I pushed my fear aside and gave it all to my heavenly Father, and he, in turn, sat with me on that piano bench and guided me to deliver my best. Thanks, Mom!

I AM HOT!

One day in May, I went to visit my parents' home in Benton Harbor to check on things. It had only been a few months into Mom's diagnosis, and I wanted to give Dad a break and to check on things at the house. (Little did I know that these trips would become regular events.) That Sunday morning, I needed to go to the grocery store for a few things for dinner that evening, so I got Mom dressed and in the car, and we headed off.

Let me remind you that in Michigan we have a saying: "If you don't like the weather, wait five minutes." That day was one of those crazy Michigan days when you can feel the warm sun on your face, yet a light jacket was also required. I outfitted Mom in a nice pair of slacks, a fleece pullover, and a light jacket. Perfect.

I encouraged Mom to push the grocery cart while I scanned the shelves for the items I needed. I discovered that having her push the cart kept her occupied and within my line of sight. We completed shopping, checked out, and headed for the car for the return trip home.

While we were in the store, the sun had heated the car up considerably, and Mom began to complain about the warmth. I assured her that it would soon cool down and to just be patient.

Mom was always strong-willed, and waiting a few minutes for the car to cool down just was not in her nature. As I started to drive home, Mom unsnapped her seat belt, took off everything—and I mean everything—from the waist up, neatly folded them, placed them in her lap, and happily enjoyed the scenic ride home—topless.

What could I do? Pull over and dress her on the side of the road? I decided just to let her enjoy herself. If we were lucky, I could bypass all the traffic lights and stop signs to get us back home without stopping. How would I ever explain her nakedness if we got stopped? "I'm sorry, Officer. My mother decided she was too warm for clothing." Best to just keep driving.

WHAT WOULD MR. BLACKWELL SAY?

One warm weekend in July, I took a day trip to visit Mom and Dad. Mom was still living at home at the time, and I was looking forward to spending time with both of them while making sure they had everything they needed.

I found Mom sitting on the back porch on a little stool by the door, where she could enjoy a full view of the backyard and the open spaces. She sat with her legs demurely crossed, looking so comfortable and peaceful as she surveyed the neighbors' vegetable garden and fruit trees. Nothing unusual in that, but what she was wearing on this warm summer day drew me up short. Mom was going for the layered look—and then some. I can only describe it as a summer-winter-fall ensemble.

She was the lady in red, wearing a red wool blazer buttoned at the waist, her cotton pajama top peeking out from underneath. From the waist down, she sported a red plaid linen skirt, and on her feet a pair of red footie socks and her usual pair of black leather lace-up shoes. Completing the ensemble was a jaunty red flannel tam. (Sort of a French flair, I thought.)

After assessing her outfit from head to toe, I quickly turned around to hide my laugher, as well as regain my composure. Kissing her softly on the cheek, I said, "Hey, Mom. Looks like you've got a summer-winter thing going on today."

Her reply was her signature affirmation "Ah. Hmmm."

I replied, "Why don't we go inside and see what Daddy is doing?"

She took my hand and followed me into the house, and within the next couple of hours, I had her dressed into something much more comfortable and appropriate, transforming her from a candidate for Mr. Blackwell's Worst-Dressed List.

YIKES! DAD IS WEARING MOM'S PANTS!

One of my usual visits to see my parents provided yet another story to be included in this project. I will be the first to admit that I have helped more than a few certified nursing aides realize that caregiving may not be the right career choice for them and strongly encourage them to keep looking.

For example, one Saturday I made my usual visit to the facility to spend some quality time with them. A few minutes after I arrived, my dad needed assistance getting to the bathroom, and I obliged.

Dad is roughly six feet tall, weighs about 220 pounds, and wears about a size 50 pant. Miss Bee Bee was a petite four foot nine, weighed about 115 pounds, and wore a 12 petite slack. Once I got him to the bathroom, I noticed that his jeans looked different, but I was unsure how or why. But most certainly something was amiss.

Although Dad is wheelchair bound, he is able to stand and pivot to sit on the toilet. We began the process of standing, getting his balance as I brought his pants down. And there it was.

He was wearing Bee Bee's jeans! (Go ahead and laugh. I still laugh about that.)

I kept looking at him, wondering how much effort it took to shove all of who he is into such a small space. I looked at him and then back at Bee Bee's pants. I asked myself, "How long did that take?" Honestly, my mother's pants looked like tights on my dad. I turned to my dad and said, "Hey there, do you know that you have on Mom's jeans?"

He replied, "I thought something felt different, but I wasn't sure. Thank goodness you stopped by." You think?

I called for the nursing aide who had dressed him that morning and inquired, "How did this happen?" She, unfortunately, did not have an answer. Therefore, I wished her the best of luck on her next assignment, and that was the end of that.

DRIVING MISS BEE BEE

Apart from removing her clothing, Mom was a great passenger in the car. When she, Dad, and I were out together, she sat comfortably in the middle of the back seat, alert to everything around her. She never napped or needed entertainment. In fact, she was very helpful. How? She read aloud every single traffic or street sign we pass. For example:

"Slow traffic ahead."
"Speed limit fifty-five."
"Merge left."
"Stop."
"Truck crossing."
"Left turn only."
"Road work ahead."

Now if Mom had been a toddler learning to read, this might have been cute or even entertaining for a mile or two. But just imagine taking her on a 280-mile road trip to Ohio to visit my sister. There were times when I thought I would rather put a needle in my eye than listen to her say, "Passing zone ahead" for the umpteenth time. She never missed a sign. Ever. She read them all aloud. Every. Single. One. To make matters worse, Dad, who sat in the front passenger seat, would goad her on by pointing to a sign. Instantly, Mom would call it out from the back seat, which would make Dad chuckle and brought a smile to my face. He found it endearing instead of annoying, and that makes me grateful for this time when we could laugh and enjoy our time together as a family.

SERVICE CENTER 2

To begin, first I'd like to offer my apologies to the great state of Ohio and specifically the women in the restroom of Service Center 2 on the 80/90 toll road between Toledo and Cleveland.

One weekend in the summer of 2005, we decided to take a ride to Cleveland to see my sister and her family. At the time, it seemed like a good idea—a chance for us to spend time together as my niece was also getting baptized that Sunday.

To orchestrate such a trip requires careful thought and advanced planning, so I started right away to set things in order. I rented a minivan that had a DVD player, made hotel reservations, arranged a sitter for my dog, and prepared snacks for the 280-mile drive.

So far, so good. It was a beautiful day for driving, and we— Mom, Dad, and my husband—left home right on schedule.

We agreed to stop about every ninety minutes to stretch our legs and to take bathroom breaks. When you are traveling with older people, this is a requirement clearly stated in the "Traveling with Old People" rule book. For the first two stops, everything went according to the book.

Once we left Michigan and got on the turnpike in Ohio, our destination was just two hours away. I popped a movie in the DVD player for Mom and Dad to enjoy. There they were in the back seat, holding hands as if they were at a drive-in movie theatre—a Kodak moment for sure.

We were right on schedule when we pulled into a service center to take our last biological break—and that is where my careful planning fell apart. As we had done on previous breaks, my husband and father headed to the men's restroom, and I took Mom into the ladies' room. I always headed for the larger, roomier handicapped stall so that we could share the space as we went about our business, if you know what I mean.

Mom was at a point in her disease where she could still toilet herself without assistance. However, some prompting was needed so that we could avoid accidents. Once in the stall, I encouraged her to go. She replied with a resounding "No!" So, having to go myself, I decided to demonstrate by example, during which Mom unlocked the stall door and flung it open. There I was on full display. I quickly reached for the door to pull it shut, but it was out of reach. Now I was multitasking: trying to finish my business with an audience a few feet away and close the door, keep Mom contained, and convince her to use the facilities as she argued back. It sounded something like this:

Mom (yelling): "Stop. Let go of me."

Me (loudly whispering): "Mom, please sit down."

Mom (shouting loudly): "You're hurting me."

Me (whispering louder): "You have to sit down."

Me (now hissing like a snake): "Mom, please!"

As I was confined to the stall, I had no idea how many women heard us, but I'm sure they were becoming concerned—for who, I don't know. One way or another, there was going to be a scene—either me with my pants down chasing Mom around the restroom, or a report of elder abuse.

Finally, I relented and allowed her to exit the handicap stall—upon which she immediately dashed into the adjacent stall and locked the door. Right about this time, I noticed the look of shock and awe on the faces of the other travelers watching this situation. Several thoughts went through my mind. *Maybe I can just leave her here and pick her up on the way back. Perhaps one of these women could take her for the weekend.* But I dismissed both notions when my beloved mother simply took care of her business, exited the stall, washed her hands, and said to me, "Okay, honey, let's go!"

Just to be clear, I assured all the onlookers that she indeed belonged to me and all was well. I am still not certain that they actually believed me, but one very kind lady quietly said, "Bless you."

IT IS JUST ONE OF THOSE DAYS!

Before I had to move Mom to an assisted living facility in Grand Rapids so she would be closer to me to help take care of her, she lived at home with my dad. For more than a year, I would travel every other weekend to check on them and take care of things around their house.

Both my parents took great pride in the appearance of their home. Not only was everything neat and tidy, but the laundry and grocery shopping were completed on a regular schedule. But as Mom's illness progressed, things started to slip, so I would alternate weekends, taking care of either my own household or the things I needed to do to keep things afloat there.

I made the trek early Saturday morning to get a jump start on their housework. It was a beautiful, sunny July day, and I looked forward to spending time with both of them. When I arrived, Dad was always so relieved to see me, and it was disheartening to see the growing fatigue on his face from trying to manage Mom in whatever state she was in, as well as keep the household organized.

During this time, Mom was still able to dress herself (sometimes in fascinating clothing choices) and do some household chores. Unfortunately, she was often unable to complete what she started. For example, she would start doing the dishes but not quite finish. Or perhaps she would go into a bedroom for whatever reason and get distracted with an item on the dresser. People with dementia exhibit the same behavior many times over. I likened it to a needle

37

on a record that would get stuck and keep repeating, over and over, until you gave it a gentle nudge. In these moments, Mom needed a nudge to get her to move onto another activity.

On this particular Saturday, she was still in her pajamas from the night before, so my first task was to see if I could get her cleaned up and into something more appropriate for the day. But she was in her no phase, so I decided to leave her alone for the time being as I went about my to-do list.

I started to vacuum and dust as usual, while Dad retreated to his little home office to play games on his computer. This was his respite time, and I certainly wanted him to enjoy the solitude. Because things were relatively quiet, I thought it would be a great day to move furniture around and do some deep cleaning. So that's what I did. I was multitasking in high gear as I had many little projects going on at once—a load of laundry in the washing machine, cleaning products were strewn about, and a collection of dirty dishes in the sink.

I was about two hours into my cleaning routine when the doorbell rang. Immediately I thought, *Heaven's sake. Not a good time for company!* The furniture was in disarray, nothing was back in its usual place, and I was not prepared to entertain anyone as I had a schedule to keep. My dog, which I brought along to keep Dad company, alerted by the doorbell, began barking and running around. But most of all, my mother was not properly dressed. In fact, she had somehow slipped away and put her underwear—bra and panties—on the outside of her yellow silk pajamas!

I tried to see who was at the door without being seen, but it was a failed attempt at being inconspicuous. There's nothing I could do at this point but take a deep breath and open the door to my father's friends: members of the Jehovah Witnesses church making their weekly visit. Dad loved these regular conversations, as he has always been a student of the Bible and appreciated a healthy debate of comparing religions. I greeted them, led them to the living room, and left to get Dad.

While all this was going on, Mom was calmly standing at the dining table thumbing through a sales flyer from the day's papers. She acted as if she had never heard the doorbell, and she never looked up to see who was entering the house to see her remarkable ensemble on full display. I remember thinking, *Well, there's nothing I can do about that now, is there?*

Fortunately, Dad's guests were very polite and understanding. They were aware of Mom's condition and never batted an eye but greeted her with a little wave and a warm hello. But I bet they had a story to tell once they finished their visit. I only hope they threw in a little prayer at the end.

YOUR DENTURES ARE WHERE?

My parents and I were traveling to Princeton, West Virginia, to attend my uncle's funeral. We thought it best to fly down instead of driving twelve hundred miles. The largest airport to Princeton was Charleston, West Virginia, about ninety-three miles due north. I made our plane reservations and informed the airlines that I would be traveling with two seniors who needed assistance on each leg of the trip. I rented a full-size car, reserved two hotel rooms, and notified the family that we would be arriving the day before the funeral. I was quite confident that I had all my bases covered and was up to the challenge of handling this trip on my own.

Again, because Benton Harbor has no airport, instead, this time, we were flying out of Grand Rapids, a little more than an hour away. We were on an early-morning flight, which meant that I was up at least three hours before our departure time to ensure that we arrived early enough to get through security, check our luggage, and take a quick biological break before boarding the plane. So far, so good.

We arrived at the gate in plenty of time and were allowed to board before the other passengers, giving me time to get my parents seated and buckled in. Now, for Dad, this was an easy and quick task to do. No problem. However, Miss Bee Bee decided to sit on her seat belt and would not get up so I could buckle it. She went completely in her no phase, refusing to stand up. I was standing in the aisle, reaching over Dad, who was seated in the aisle seat, trying to get the seat belt out from under Mom. I looked like I was auditioning

41

for Cirque du Soleil. My butt—not that it's unusually large—was blocking the aisle. Other passengers were starting to board the plane, and clearly, I was holding them up. I pleaded with Mom (or maybe swore at her) to get up. Finally, between Dad and me, we got her buckled in and settled. I took my seat in the row directly behind them and fell asleep before we even took off.

We had an hour layover between the first and second leg of the trip, which gave me just enough time to get them a snack, take a bathroom break, and make our way to our next departure gate. The two wheelchairs I ordered were waiting for us at the arrival gate, along with two airport employees to push them, as I could not have managed pushing both of them through the airport. We rolled through the crowds without any difficulties whatsoever, arriving at our departure gate with time to spare. Again, we boarded before the other passengers and headed to our seats. Mom took her seat by the window, and Dad sat down beside her. Although she had been on another plane just an hour before, she broke into tears, babbling about being afraid to fly and wanting to get off the plane. Exhausted, I looked at Daddy and simply said, "Deal with that." I sat down directly behind them and went to sleep. Somehow, he managed to calm her, and we arrived without incident, safe, sound, and on schedule, with only a short two-hour drive between us and our final destination.

We flew into the Yeager Airport in Charleston, West Virginia. It is a nice-sized airport, but it did not have a Jetway to connect the plane to the terminal. Therefore, we walked down a set of stairs to deplane and then walked to the terminal to the baggage claim, moving slowly as it had been quite a long day already.

After we retrieved our luggage, we headed to the car rental counter. Dad was holding Mom's hand so she would not wander away. We were treated with real southern hospitality as the rental agent offered to bring our car to the terminal doors instead of having us walk to the lot across the street. It was either southern hospitality or because I looked like a pack mule, dragging my luggage and theirs through the terminal.

After loading them and our luggage in the car and getting everyone's seat belt fastened, I got behind the wheel for the ninety-minute drive to our hotel in Princeton and realized that all I had eaten all day was airplane peanuts and I needed to get something substantial to eat before I passed out.

Dad responded with "There's a restaurant right next door to where we will be staying." I just gave him one of my "Are you out of your mind?" looks. He meekly responded with "Or we could get something nearby."

I turned to the back seat to check on Mom one more time—and did a double take. When we had left Michigan, her dentures were firmly in place, but now they were gone! I looked at her and then gazed out on the runway. Could they be on the plane? If they were, they'd just have to stay there, because I was not getting out of the car. *Well, some flight attendant is in for a surprise*, I thought as I pulled out of the parking lot.

After twelve hours of travel and more than a few challenges, we arrived at the hotel and checked into our rooms across the hall from each other. I got Mom and Dad settled, ordered their dinner, and went to my room to unpack and enjoy a few moments of alone time before returning to help Dad get Mom ready for bed.

Unfortunately, I made the poor decision to lie down for just a few minutes, which turned into an hour because I fell asleep. I awoke with a start and hurried to their room—which was a complete disaster. Mom had completely rearranged the furniture, the bedding, and anything else she could move. Daddy, dressed in his pajamas, was nestled under the covers, watching the local news. He was the calm in the middle of the storm. It took about an hour, but I finally got Mom dressed for bed and tucked in.

Before I returned to my room, I told Dad I would return in the morning to get her dressed for the service and down to breakfast. With my hand on the doorknob, I said, "Oh, one more thing. I gave her a sleeping pill so she won't wake up in the middle of the night and not know where she is."

He asked, "You gave her a sleeping pill?"

"Yes," I said.

He replied, "So did I." We looked at each other and burst into laughter, as Mom lay there sleeping, totally oblivious to us.

Needless to say, we all got a well-deserved and peaceful, uninterrupted rest that night. And by the way, her dentures were in her purse.

DO NOT LET THEM RUN
AROUND NAKED

If your loved one is having difficulty with getting dressed, then try one of these tried-and-true techniques.

1. Consider buying clothing void of prints, patterns or intricate designs. Your loved one may become mesmerized and fascinated by colors and shapes. The more decorative the clothing item is, the more difficult it will be to get your loved one dressed.

2. Rearrange closets and dresser drawers so that coordinating shirts, tops, pants, and skirts are hung as outfits together, which will help expedite dressing in the morning by eliminating searching for tops and bottoms that match.

3. Create wardrobe choices so that everything is interchangeable. This will save valuable time and energy on those days when the patient is agitated or easily irritated.

4. Avoid clothing that has buttons, zippers, or snaps. You will want to invest in elastic waistbands, pullover tops, and Velcro shoes.

5. If your loved one needs assistance with toileting, use this time to dress or even undress them. You will kill two birds with one stone.

6. If your loved one lives in a care facility, remember to label all clothes with their name. This helps to insure the items get returned correctly from laundry services.

7. Gripper socks like those worn in hospitals help guard against falls. Consider having an inventory of several pairs on hand.

8. "Older is colder." Always have a sweater or jacket handy. Body temperatures in the elderly are usually colder than in the average adult.

9. Check regularly for fluctuations in weight gain or loss to make sure their clothing still fits properly.

ISN'T MAIL TAMPERING A FEDERAL OFFENSE?

People who have dementia will often leave their homes and wander away. We all have seen news reports about such things happening. Today, there are many devices available, ranging from simple to complicated, to help keep loved ones safe if they wander.

Mom's identification device was rather simple: an ID bracelet with the Alzheimer's symbol on it, a toll-free phone number, her first name, and her ID number. She believed it was her watch, and we chose not to tell her anything different.

As a part of her daily routine, Mom would go to the mailbox located at the end of our hundred-foot-long driveway to collect the mail. No harm in that, right? Each day she would come into the house with an armful of assorted envelopes, magazines, and a variety of weekly newspapers. I would think, *Wow, must be a heavy mail delivery day.*

One day, I decided to take a closer look and discovered that most of this mail was not addressed to her and Dad. Instead, it was addressed to the neighbors whose last names were Emerson, Boone, Browning, or Roberts. Yep, Mom was a mail thief. At last recollection, the post office takes a very dim view with tampering with the US mail, and there could be serious consequences.

Then I thought, *When did she do this? When did she turn to a life of crime? I was in the house the whole time and never saw or heard her leave.* Then I discovered how she was doing it. In spite of her age and her condition, she was as stealthy as a cat. She would slip on her quiet rubber-soled shoes, slip out the back door, make her way through the fruit trees that lined the property, and head for the road.

What could I do? I loaded Mom into my car along with the bundles of mail, and as discreetly as I could, we rode down our road and redelivered the mail to its rightful owners. And did she learn her lesson? No! A few days later, it would happen all over again. I became a familiar sight on the mail route as I played postman for my mother, the mail thief.

SHOULD A NIECE TALK TO
HER UNCLE THAT WAY?

When Mom was still living at home and still quite ambulatory, nearly each day she would venture one and a half miles down the road to her brother Bob's house. The houses were on a partially paved road that saw little traffic. Fortunately, the road between the two houses was a straight shot, so if I went looking for Mom, all I had to do was look down the road, where I could clearly see her in the distance on the way to Bob's.

As a bit of a curmudgeon, Uncle Bob did not have an open-door policy, and I'm fairly certain Mom showed up without an invitation. She never stayed long, but she always managed to annoy him. On this autumn day, however, whatever she did pushed him over the edge.

Daddy called to tell me that Uncle Bob had called him to complain that Mom would come in and rearrange things—go through the kitchen cabinets, open doors, and just basically interrupt his solitude—and he'd had enough. If she showed up again, he would lock her out of the house—no ifs, ands, or buts. Dad tried to explain that he tried to keep an eye on Mom but that she would simply slip out the door and walk to Bob's.

Hearing the sheer exhaustion in Dad's voice, I decided that it was time for my only remaining living uncle and I to have a chat— Cheryl style. So I called him.

My uncle repeated the same story he'd told Dad, basically accusing Mom of invading his privacy. I listened to him rant and rave, and then it was my turn.

I explained to my beloved uncle Bob that Dad did not "send" her down to his house and that she had no control over her uninvited visits. "The next time she comes over," I said, "just call Dad, and he will come pick her up."

But I wasn't finished. Furthermore, I told my uncle that because he was my mother's older brother, I expected him to watch out for her and help keep her safe. I expected him to protect her and help my dad to keep her safe. Until the time that her disease progressed and we would have to move her to a facility for the rest of her life, we would continue to care for her at home.

Then, as firmly—but respectfully—as I could, I told Uncle Bob that if I *ever* heard about him even talking about locking *my* mother out of anybody's house, he would experience the wrath of Cheryl, unlike anything he had experienced before.

But I could stay angry for only so long. As only my uncle Bob could do, he melted my heart when he said, "No, niecy, you know I wouldn't do anything to hurt her, but ..." His voice trailed off. My voice softened as I wished him well, letting him know that I would check on him next time I was in town.

Later that day, I got a second call from my dad asking me simply, "Cheryl, what did you say to Bob?"

Let's just say the subject of locking Mom out of Uncle Bob's house never came up again.

AUNT SUE'S FUNERAL

My mother's sister, Sue, was five years older than Mom, and the two were as different as night and day. Although both women were well educated, devoted community volunteers, and loving mothers, Aunt Sue enjoyed being in the spotlight, aspired to be successful, and loved being recognized for her successes. In contrast, Mom was humble, preferred to be behind the scenes, and didn't seek out attention or accolades. However, there was no doubt that Mom loved Sue unconditionally and supported her no matter what situation presented itself.

For several years, our families lived just a few houses from each other, and we enjoyed each other's company almost on a daily basis until our family moved to the country some six miles away. After many years, Aunt Sue and her husband divorced, and she moved to Florida, where she lived for about twenty years until 2004, when a major stroke required her daughter, Renee, to move her into a skilled nursing facility in Ann Arbor, Michigan.

On December 12, 2005, Aunt Sue passed away peacefully with her two children and granddaughter at her bedside. Although my aunt and I had a somewhat adversarial relationship, I was saddened by her passing because I knew that my mother would be upset.

The family hour was on a Friday night at the funeral home. Most of our family and extended family made the trip to pay their respects. Regardless of our differences, we are a close-knit group and always support each other. We had not been together for a while, so far from being a solemn affair, there was laughter and talking as we caught up with each other.

At the front of the chapel, Aunt Sue was lying in state in an open casket. I was seated in the back of the chapel talking with family, when one of my cousins came to me and said with alarm, "Cheryl, Aunt Bee Bee is walking toward the casket. What should we do?"

I replied, "That's okay. She can go, but I think you should go with her." (Let's just say I don't do well at funerals.)

In true Miss Bee Bee style, Mom strutted up the aisle to the front of the chapel. When she reached the casket, she stretched out her arms and placed her hands on its side. We all held our collective breath as she looked her sister up and down, down and up. She then said, "Well, that is Sue all right, but I did not think I would see her like this!" Then she simply turned around and walked back down the aisle.

That's one way to close down a visitation.

The service was held the next morning at the Episcopalian church my aunt attended. It was a lovely service and a very warm and appropriate remembrance of Aunt Sue—even if the priest did refer to her by the wrong name: Helen. I'm sure there were a few stifled giggles from the other guests as we in unison reminded him, "Her name was Sue."

He responded, "Sorry, I was thinking about my wife." Why? Was she dead too? Who knows?

The service included Holy Communion. Each guest rose, walked to the communion rail at the front of the church, knelt on a padded kneeler, received the host, and then rose and returned to their seat.

Aunt Sue's immediate family was seated on the first pew, with the rest of the family, including Mom and Dad, seated directly behind them. I sat in the pew behind Mom and Dad to keep an eye on Mom.

As I approached the communion rail, from the pews I heard Mom loudly whisper to Dad, "Alfred, isn't that Cheryl? Where is she going with those noisy shoes?" Daddy attempted to keep her quiet, but to no avail. As I knelt, I glanced her way and gave her the eye. I didn't dare look over my shoulder to see the reactions from family and friends.

Mom settled down, and the service continued without further interruption—or giggles.

THE TURNING POINT

As Mom's illness progressed, Dad grew into his role as her caregiver, managing as best he could. For nearly five years, I drove to their house every two weeks to give him a much-needed break. When it could be arranged, I would bring them to spend the weekend with my husband, Larry, and me so Dad could truly relax as I looked out for Mom.

Such was my plan on Labor Day weekend, 2005. The weather was beautiful, so we decided to spend time outdoors, gardening and sitting on the deck that stretched nearly the entire length of our house, which Larry and I designed to accommodate family and friends for large gatherings. It was situated on nearly an acre lot surrounded by old, hundred-foot-tall trees. We both love flower gardening, and together we transformed our backyard into a colorful collection of perennials that bloomed from spring through fall.

Larry, like my dad, was the chef of the family and grew spices and herbs in pots that lined one end of the deck. Since this was going to be the last cookout for the summer, Larry was grilling a variety of barbecue meats and roasting corn for dinner. The fresh aroma of a good home-cooked meal filled the kitchen, making us eager to sit down and enjoy Larry's culinary masterpiece.

Mom and I were pulling weeds from the flower beds and trimming back perennials in anticipation of the coming winter months. As we worked, my best friend, Mattie, stopped by for a visit and to enjoy time with my folks. I reveled in spending time outdoors on autumn days like these. In a short time, we would all be confined to the house for the next five months, battling our merciless Michigan winters.

We finished our work outside just as dinner was ready, I asked Larry and Mattie to keep a watch on Mom for a few minutes while I got cleaned up. Although she was aging, she moved fast and always found something to get into that she shouldn't. I assured them I would shower quickly.

I had barely gotten covered with soap when my husband popped his head around the shower curtain, asking me if I was going to be much longer. I replied, "No, why do you ask?"

He replied, "Well, your mom got into the garage and fell. I think her leg is broken."

I jumped out of the shower, grabbed my robe, and ran to the garage, leaving a trail of suds and water behind me. There she was on the floor of the garage wincing with pain. Apparently Mom was going to let our dog outside and missed a step as she entered the garage. Mattie was with her, trying to keep her calm and still. Once I arrived, Mattie ran inside to get an ice pack as Larry gently picked her up and carried her to the sofa, and I called an ambulance.

And where was Dad while all this commotion was happening? If you recall, Labor Day weekend, 2005, was the same weekend that Hurricane Katrina ravaged New Orleans and parts of Mississippi, and he was seated smack in front of our TV with his back to us, completely mesmerized by the continuous coverage of the disaster on CNN. Now you need to know that my parents did not have cable or satellite TV at their home, so whenever they visited, Dad spent hours exploring all that cable TV had to offer. He was totally riveted by the images on TV.

Once I got off the phone with 911, I tapped Dad on the shoulder to tell him that I was going with Mom to the hospital, because she had fallen and her leg was possibly broken. He looked up at me and said, "Oh. Are we going to eat dinner first?" I walked away.

Once the paramedics arrived, they were very kind and gentle with her. Mom basked in all the attention, and I think she was even flirting a bit. Two paramedics checked her vitals while asking her questions to determine her pain level as three volunteer paramedics observed and took notes.

We got her loaded into the ambulance and made our way to the hospital without incident. I rode along in the ambulance, and Mattie and Dad followed closely behind. Mom could see Dad through the back window of the ambulance and asked who that woman with her husband was. The paramedics and I laughed, relieved that the pain medicine seemed to be working. Larry remained behind in case I needed something from home.

As we drove to the hospital, I began to wonder what would happen next. Perhaps the accident was a sign that the time had come for us to realize that Mom could not return home and be cared for by Dad. This injury, now coupled with the progression of her dementia, meant that it was time for her to move to a secured dementia facility.

Once we arrived at the hospital, Mom was seen by a very handsome young doctor who exhibited warmth and sincerity toward her. His calm demeanor reassured me that we would survive this ordeal. Kindly, he asked how she broke her leg. Flirtatiously, she replied, "I jumped off the porch!" His eyes widened as he looked at me for either confirmation or an explanation.

As I stood in the emergency room, I knew that the next few days would be an emotional roller coaster unlike anything I ever faced. In addition to coping with her broken leg, I knew it was time to make the call I'd been dreading: the call to make arrangements to move her to the memory-loss care facility I had chosen when she was first diagnosed.

Making such decisions is the ultimate challenge for a caregiver. I knew that my family trusted my research and my instincts, but I had my doubts about my ability to make the best choice for Miss Bee Bee. "One step at a time," I told myself. I took a deep breath and slowly exhaled.

Another new chapter had just begun.

MOM'S NEW HOME

On Friday, September 9, 2005, just a few days after that glorious Labor Day weekend when all seemed right with the world, I moved Mom from her home in Benton Harbor to a secured dementia facility in Grand Rapids, about three miles from where I worked. The timing could not have been worse in terms of having help from my family.

Dad, still reeling from the events over the weekend, refused to come back to Grand Rapids to help, as he blamed me for Mom's accident and accused me of planning not to take them back home that weekend, and that I had been plotting for months to relocate them both closer to me. Of course, I knew that he did not mean what he said, but it still hurt. We both needed time to let this moment pass and forgive his hurtful words, so I turned all my energies to Mom's new living arrangements.

I can usually rely on my husband and my sister, Lisa, but both are school teachers, and it was the start of the school year. Therefore, I was left on my own to get this done. Lisa knew how difficult this would be for me and sent me a beautiful bouquet of flowers to lift my spirits.

I was filled with emotion and uncertainty as I packed up Mom's clothes and toiletries and got her dressed in a beautiful new outfit. The facility was a lovely place situated on a small lake circled by lots of trees. Her room faced the lake, where she could enjoy watching the swans and ducks splash about in the water. Her room, like all of the others, was furnished with a bed, a dresser, a large, comfortable chair, and a private bathroom.

Families were encouraged to bring familiar and comforting personal items to add a homey touch, but I had brought only a few photographs. A few months later, Lisa did her "Martha Stewart" thing by adding pictures, a small sofa, a TV, and other accessories to make Mom's room inviting and homelike. She did a great job because any time we were visiting, inevitably one of us would fall asleep on the sofa. Mission accomplished.

After I unpacked her clothes, put her toiletries away, got Mom settled into her room, and completed the intake paperwork with the administration, I knew it was time for me to depart, but I was uncertain how to leave. Apparently the staff, sensing my distress, simply took Mom aside and started talking to her and finding ways to occupy her so I could slip out the door. I half expected Mom to come running out the door pleading to come with me—not to leave her there. If she did, I would have taken her back home with me and tried the next day. Mercifully, that did not happen. I asked staff to call me if there were any problems, and I walked out the door.

Tears flooded my eyes as I drove away with a deep pain piercing my chest. I knew I had no choice and that this was the best decision given the current situation. I reminded myself of all the things I had learned about Mom's disease and that she needed the extra help that we, as her family, could no longer provide. I assured myself that I would see her every day to make sure she was doing all right; after all, my office was just a quick five-minute drive away.

Once the facility was out of sight, I needed to go somewhere to allow me to regain my composure and relax a bit before heading home. Retail therapy was in order, and the mall was just around the corner. After walking around for a while, I headed home so that I could just sit quietly and reflect on the events of the past week. I sat on the deck where just eight days ago Mom and I had worked in the flower beds, laughing and talking.

I struggled with the fact that Mom was surrounded by unfamiliar faces, living in a place that would be her home until the day she passed. I thought about Dad living alone for the first time in fifty-plus years marriage. I knew that neighbors would stop by and check on him and that he could now go out and do some of the things he enjoyed the most without worry. Best of all, he could rest.

Mom adjusted amazingly well to life in the assisted living facility. I did not get a call from the staff that weekend, so I was anxious to see how she was getting along. During my lunch break on Monday, I went to visit. As it was lunchtime, the staff was setting the tables as residents slowly made their way to the dining room. I scanned the room anxiously, looking for her, and soon saw her walking right toward me. She looked up and said, "Hi, Cheryl," and kept on walking as if she had been there her whole life. She sat down at the table and started a conversation with the other ladies seated near her. A weight lifted off my shoulders as I finally felt like I had made the right choice for her care.

BUSY MISS BEE BEE

Before her illness, Mom was the assistant director of the Benton Harbor Housing Commission and lived in a house that had five bedrooms and two bathrooms. Never the type to just sit still, she was always finding something to do, whether cleaning out drawers, rearranging closets, moving furniture, and such. There had been laundry to do, groceries to purchase, and a family to care for. Now that she was living in an assisted living facility, it would be easy to imagine her being bored to tears. Quite the contrary! Now she had twenty bedrooms to keep her busy. And she certainly was busy! Residents would return to their rooms to find their dresser drawers emptied, closets rearranged, and even their bedding topsy-turvy.

And because she had worked outside the home as a professional administrator, she was very comfortable in an office environment. Therefore, it should not have come as a surprise when one day I walked in to find her sitting at the nurse's station with a pad of paper and pencil, seemingly working on something. I watched her for a few minutes, amused by her intensity of focus. She appeared happy and content in this somewhat familiar office environment as I watched with amusement. After all, what harm was she doing? I soon had my answer.

A few minutes into my visit, the phone at the reception desk rang, and before I knew it, Mom answered it! "Hello. Yes. No, they're not here." And she promptly hung up. I moved closer to her and asked Mom what she was doing. She said innocently, "I am doin' my work." Then she proceeded to scribble something on her scratch pad.

To this day, I have no idea who was on the other end of the line. I gently convinced her that work was over and walked her back to her room.

MA'AM, PLEASE STEP
OUT OF THE CAR

Eventually, the time came to move Mom to a secured dementia assisted living center. Dad continued living in the home my parents had owned for more than forty years. They were separated by about seventy-five miles.

One Saturday, I wanted to drive to Dad's for the day to check on things and decided to take Mom with me. At this stage, Mom enjoyed riding in cars and being outside. Moreover, I knew how much the visit would mean to my dad and his well-being.

Once we arrived, Mom acted as if she had never moved away. She immediately began cleaning and picking up. She seemed so happy and content as she busied herself with sweeping, dusting, and arranging things—all the chores she routinely did when she was predementia.

Dad was glad to see us, of course, and needed the company. It had been about nine months since they had been together, and he seemed lonesome. He and I talked about the things I wanted to get done that weekend, and he was just as eager to get them done too. He was doing as well as expected living on his own. The house needed some vacuuming and dusting, but otherwise, he was keeping things in order.

Dad was becoming a little unsteady on his feet. I was concerned, but not overly so, as he had a cane to help him get around. I offered to do his grocery shopping if he felt like he could watch Mom for the next hour while I was gone, which gave him the opportunity, of course, to be the husband and look after his wife. I had a few reservations leaving him to watch after her. Although Dad was unsteady on his feet, Mom was still in great physical shape and could walk a couple of miles without breaking a sweat.

That Saturday was a wonderful day. We enjoyed a good meal at the kitchen table, all the bills were paid and mailed, the laundry was done and put away, the house was fresh and clean, and plenty of meals were prepared for Dad to enjoy throughout the week.

Finally, it was time for Mom and me to head back to her new home. Leaving Dad alone at the home they once shared was always emotionally difficult, even under the best of circumstances. I knew he wanted us to stay longer or even have Mom return home permanently, but he and I knew that was not possible.

We got Mom in the car and safely buckled in. Dad thanked me over and over again for my help, as I promised him that we would come back very soon. Then we drove off. Even though I was only driving about ninety minutes away, I always fought back tears as we were going. Dad always walked us to the car and remained in the driveway until we were out of sight. This day would be no different.

The return trip back was pretty uneventful. Mom entertained me with her stories and anything she could see from her car window (including those darn road signs). Exhausted, I drove quietly, listening to her chatter. Soon, we were less than a half mile from Mom's residence, which was clearly visible from the intersection as I drove through it on what I could have sworn was a green light—or so I told the police officer who, red and blue lights flashing, pulled us over.

As I pulled over and put the car in park, I explained to Mom that this would only take a second, but she hardly noticed. Instead, she was completely mesmerized by the marvelous light show reflecting off the front windshield of the car. Red. Blue. Red. Blue. She never noticed the officer approaching my car or heard our conversation.

The officer asked where I was headed, and as a responsible citizen (that light was green!), I told him that my mother lived at the nearby assisted living facility and I was taking her back. It turned out that he was all too familiar with the facility because the police station was just two driveways east, and he sometimes responded to 911 calls from residents who had gotten access to a phone and would claim to have been kidnapped.

Now, it is common knowledge that you stay seated in the car unless you are asked to step out. When the officer asked for my driver's license and registration, I had to explain that my billfold was in the rear of my vehicle because Mom tended to take things out of it and hide them. He allowed me to step out of the car and open the hatch.

I unlocked the hatch from inside the car, but when I got to the back of the car and tried to raise the hatch, it was locked, so I returned to the driver's door to unlock it. Again, I tried lifting the hatch, and once again it was locked. Feeling a little frustrated and starting to panic, I said to the officer, "Let me try again. I know I unlocked it."

After the third try, the officer suggested that perhaps Mom, sitting quietly in the front passenger seat, was locking the trunk as I walked back to open it, and I wouldn't be able to hear the "thunk" over the noise of our running cars. To confirm his suspicions, he stood by the open driver's door while I walked to the back, and then hit the button to unlock the trunk. Almost immediately, we heard the second "thunk." Upon hearing the unlocking sound, Mom would press the button on her armrest, locking all the doors, including the trunk. Although she often did this while riding in the car, it never crossed my mind that she would do it while we were parked.

Both the officer and I could not contain ourselves. We laughed so hard and shook our heads at Mom's antics. What else could we do? He saw the embarrassment and stress on my face and was so patient and understanding. He let me off with a warning to be careful at that intersection because drivers often jump that traffic light and there had been some terrible accidents. He then did something most other officers wouldn't do. He told me to take care and offered a blessing for the great responsibility that I had. I expressed my heartfelt appreciation for his understanding and promised to heed his advice.

Within the next sixty seconds, I had Mom back at her place safe and sound. Proceeding carefully through the intersection, I headed home to enjoy an adult beverage and reflect on yet another Miss Bee Bee moment that would make me laugh and smile for many days to come.

SANITY TIPS FOR SUCCESSFUL ROAD TRIPS

- Anticipate, plan, and plan again. You must have a schedule so you need to know what needs to be done and when. Remember that the person you are caring for will have plans of his or her own (which may have nothing to do with what's truly going on), so be flexible and think three steps ahead.
- Always, always, always have an extra set of keys on you at all times. Inevitably you will be locked out of your own house or your own car! (If you doubt me, read Ma'am Please Step Out of the Car.)
- Keep magazines handy, especially ones with colorful pictures. Travel magazines are a wonderful source of entertainment.
- Music is therapeutic, especially if it is familiar and of their generation. This is especially true during change of seasons, weather, or other environmental changes. Play it. Sing it. Listen to it. It can help during car rides, plane rides, or any event that may lead to agitation.
- Keep a notepad with you or record reminders in a fashion where you can quickly retrieve them. Remember—you are caring for someone who cannot help to remind you that their meds are due precisely at 3:00 p.m. Write things down.
- A durable power of attorney and health care proxy are the legal documents that grant you authority to make decisions for those who cannot decide for themselves. Keep originals

in a safe place, and carry copies with you just in case something unexpected occurs.

- Remember carrying a diaper bag when your children were infants? One for an incontinent adult is not much different. Include rubber gloves, incontinence products, bags for disposal, disinfectant cloths, and an extra pair of slacks/ pants.

- A lightweight wheelchair can be a lifesaver. Get one that collapses easily for storing in a trunk of a car. Many come with a carrying bag and foot pedals and typically weigh about five pounds. They are available at most drugstores or big box stores.

THIS PLACE IS A MESS!

I am my mother's daughter, in that she and I both enjoy shopping. Before her illness, she and I would go out together on Saturdays to run errands. I enjoyed our time together immensely. Mom was entertaining and always made me laugh. We would be in and out of stores most of the morning, then stop and have a quick bite to eat before I took her back home. I decided that this tradition should continue, regardless of her mental state.

I was in the market for a new bedroom dresser, so I decided one of our stops would be a stroll through a furniture store. I picked up Mom midmorning, and off we went. It was a beautiful spring day with clear skies and warm enough for just a light jacket.

I parked the car, and we went into the large, two-story store where I had bought furniture before. Typically, Mom reached for my hand when we started walking, and today was no different. She started to describe all the things she saw, and I acknowledged with a mindless, "Hmmm."

We meandered around the store, just taking our time until one striking dresser caught my eye, and I decided to take a closer look. As sales associates approached me and asked if I needed help, I decided to let go of Mom's hand and allow her to wander on her own. How much trouble could she get into? I felt comfortable with her exploring unchaperoned.

As the sales associate and I discussed the dresser (which was on sale for a great price), I glanced around for Mom. I had lost sight of her, but since she is only four foot nine, it was not hard to do.

As I scanned the showroom, I kept hearing a noise in the distance that sounded like bubble wrap popping. I thought it best to excuse myself from the sales associate and find Mom. At last, I saw her and started walking in her direction. As I got closer, I saw that she was doing something—but what it was I couldn't figure out. Then I realized that whatever it was she was doing, it was somehow related to the "popping" sound.

Finally, she looked up and saw me. She had that wide-eyed look that suggested she was in some kind of trouble, not unlike a small child. As she quickly walked toward me, I saw she held a stack of sales tags from God-knows how many pieces of furniture and accessories. I looked at her and said, "Mom, what did you do?"

"These are everywhere!" she replied, quickly handing them to me. In doing so, she noticed another one hanging from a very attractive leather sofa.

"And there's another one!" She promptly snatched it off, snapping the plastic line that attached the tag to the sofa. Pop!

I considered trying to match the tags back to the corresponding pieces of furniture but quickly realized the futility. Either merchandise would be grossly overpriced or significantly underpriced. I returned to my friendly sales associate and apologetically gave her the tags. I tried to explain what Mom had done, as her friendly expression turned to disbelief. With that, we took our leave. I never did go back for that dresser.

BED, BATH, AND BOOM!

After the incident at the furniture store, I realized that some stores were better suited than others for my shopping excursions with Mom. Perhaps it was because the aisles were wider and there was less merchandise, quieter music, or fewer people. None of these attributes apply to my favorite store that carries a variety of home goods and unique home décor items. Displays reach to the ceiling, there are enough plates, silverware and glassware for a ten-course meal for one hundred, and of course, there are gadgets galore. I should have known better than to take her there.

I was looking forward to leisurely exploring the merchandise with Mom, but things started to go downhill the moment we walked in. We struggled over which way our cart should go, which aisles I wanted go down, or what merchandise I wanted to take a closer look at. She was becoming increasingly agitated and more difficult to redirect, so I quickly made my selections and headed to the closest register.

Once in line, it was always a challenge to hang on to Mom *and* write a check. I was unsuccessful as she finally broke free and made a beeline to the lawn chairs on display near the checkout lanes. She promptly sat in one and made herself at home, crossing her arms and legs, looking as if she was planning on staying for a while.

I quickly wrote my check and handed it to the cashier, who said it would take a minute to process. I took advantage of the time to retrieve Mom. I bent down and said to her quietly, but firmly, "Get up and let's go!" She looked me right in the eye and responded with an equally firm no. What then came out of my mouth were words that a daughter should never, ever say to her mother. But I did and will apologize to Jesus my first day in heaven.

During our verbal sparring, the cashier was calling for me to return to the checkout lane. I'm afraid I lost my temper with her as well, as I told her just to sit tight and give me a minute. Mom hadn't budged one inch, and I had reached my breaking point. I grabbed her by the arm and pulled her tiny frame out of the chair, snatched my bag from the cashier, and stormed out of the door, embarrassed and distraught.

We reached the car and I struggled to open the car door while holding my bag and Mom's hand. My mother, in the most endearing voice possible, said to me, "Now, where are we going next, my darling daughter?" I thought, *Nowhere, old lady. You're going home!*

PUT IT ON MY TAB

Many, many cities now have large grocery superstores. Typically, they are open twenty-four hours a day, seven days a week, and carry just about everything from groceries and clothing to jewelry and auto supplies.

They say you should never go grocery shopping while hungry. I say I should never take Mom shopping while she's hungry. She becomes a food magnet, and there is no controlling her.

This adventure happened before Mom moved into her care facility, and she was still living at home with Dad. I was in Benton Harbor on one of my weekend visits, and I decided to take her with me to the store to pick up a few things for dinner. She happily pushed the shopping cart down the aisle, stopping every so often to chat with perfect strangers as if she knew them. For the most part, many were quite accommodating and shared a friendly exchange of pleasantries, responding with warmth and understanding. Many times, they also laid a blessing on me for doing what I was doing.

As with many large big-box stores, the challenge lay in the checkout lanes. Unloading the groceries onto the conveyor, paying, getting the bags into the cart—all while holding onto Mom—was a sight to behold. Regardless of how few items I had, using the self-checkouts was out of the question, so I proceeded to find a lane that had very few people waiting in line. My tactic was to line up in the checkout lane in this order: cart, Mom, me. I thought this would trap her between the cart and me as I checked out.

By this time, Mom was loudly complaining that she was hungry. For those of you who have toddlers, you know the feeling. And those of you with children probably greatly appreciate the no-candy lanes, where the displayed merchandise excludes candy or snacks. But no store had a "Miss Bee Bee" lane. In a flash, she grabbed a candy bar from the shelf, unwrapped it, shoved it in her mouth in just two bites, and made the wrapper disappear—all in the span of about five seconds. By this time, the cashier had processed my order and asked, "Will there be anything else?" Still in shock, I simply shook my head but was thinking, *Did anyone see what just happened?* Hearing no alarms or sirens going off, we made a mad dash for the nearest exit. Another thing to discuss with God when I get to heaven.

HELP! I'M STUCK TO A
BOX OF COOKIES

Just three years after moving Mom to the care facility in Grand Rapids, Dad could no longer care for himself, and we moved him to a skilled nursing center just four miles from Mom. On occasion, Dad would join Mom and me on our shopping excursions. It gave us time to get some fresh air and enjoy the time together.

After the chocolate bar incident, I would pick them up about midmorning after they had their breakfast. Miss Bee Bee was still walking and could do so without any assistance. Dad, however, needed one of the motorized carts that most stores have available for customer use.

Our arrival at the store was a ballet of sorts. I would pull up and park the car close to the entrance, so Dad didn't have to walk far to get to a motorized cart. Mom sat patiently in the car waiting as I got Dad settled. He would then motor into the store, promising to wait by the door while I parked and walked with Mom inside.

Once inside, we made an interesting caravan. Mom commanded her position of pushing the cart with me beside her. Dad followed at a safe distance just behind us. This day, our destination was another large specialty store, with its wide aisles, soft lighting, and minimal displays. Harsh lights, vertical displays, and narrow aisles could be overstimulating for Mom and could wake the toddler living inside her.

Dad occasionally would veer off to look around on his own, which was just fine with me. Shopping on his own gave Dad a sense of independence and confidence, and I didn't have to wonder where he was, as sooner or later we would reconnect and finish up our shopping as a family.

About twenty minutes after Dad left our group, I began hearing a noise in the distance that sounded like metal hitting metal, over and over. I didn't think much about at first until I realized that I had not seen Dad in a while. I started to backtrack to find him, unconsciously heading toward the clanging sound.

I soon found him a few aisles away, seemingly stuck to a display rack filled with cookies. He had tried to make a tight turn around the display, and the back of the cart got hung up on the bottom shelf of the display. He kept backing up and trying to go forward, but he could not get loose, as packages of cookies bounced off the shelves and onto the floor. As I tried to dislodge the cart and replace the cookies, Mom stood behind the cart, looking at things on the shelves and reading labels, oblivious to everything.

After all that excitement, there was no possible way to continue shopping. As we headed toward the checkout lanes, a cashier, who had witnessed our little accident, graciously waived me over to her lane. A caregiver herself, she was kind and understanding as she checked us out in record time. We performed our entrance ballet in reverse, trying to make a graceful exit.

MORE SANITY TIPS TO SUCCESSFUL CAREGIVING

It is an honor to be a caregiver. To be entrusted with the responsibility of taking care of a loved one fulfills an expectation that God has of us. "Honor your father and your mother, that your days may be long upon the land which the Lord your God is giving you." (Exodus 20:12, NKJV)

- Having said that, you are not Wonder Woman or Superman. You cannot do it all. Do not be afraid to ask for help from friends, your church, or even support groups. An Internet search for "caregiver resources" will turn up a plethora of information in your area.
- Some days you will be overwhelmed, frustrated, or angry. When you are in that state of mind, be mindful not to demean or belittle your loved one. Words like *cannot* or *do not* often diminish their self-esteem and can hurt. Use encouraging words like *try, can I do that for you*, or *you're doing great today*. Tell your loved one that he or she is beautiful/handsome. It will make him or her smile and feel special.
- Perhaps your aggravation stems from the fact that your loved one simply can't hear you. Save a lung! Change hearing aid batteries at least once a week.

- It is okay to make mistakes. Don't beat yourself up and stop trying to be an overachiever. There are times when things do not go according to plan. Let it go. You will have other opportunities for a do-over.
- Caregiving is exhausting. You cannot be effective if you are sleeping on your feet. When you get the chance, take a nap.
- Write notes and keep a to-do list. Whether you use a paper notebook, a calendar, or a smartphone or computer app, use whatever system works for you. And no matter how small or silly, if there's a chance of forgetting it, write it down. This is especially helpful when administering medicines. (Do not ask me how I know this. Just trust me.)
- As an added layer of protection for your loved one's privacy, utilize the National Do Not Call registry. This registry will block unwanted calls from telemarketers. For more information go to: www.donotcall.gov.
- And last, do not underestimate the power of prayer.

GOD KNOWS WHAT IS IN MY HEART

Both my parents were committed members of their church for many years. They tithed appropriately, volunteered when needed, and were committed to the church's doctrine. There was no reason why I couldn't continue this tradition even though my mom was now living in Grand Rapids.

I took Mom to a large, established Baptist church located in the heart of the city. I had a feeling that she would thoroughly enjoy the singing and the Spirit-filled sanctuary during the two-hour service.

Mom was still new to Grand Rapids and her new home, and on the day we went to church, she was still recovering from her broken leg. She wore a cast up to her knee and used a wheelchair to get around. We arrived at church early enough to get a seat at the end of the pew that allowed us an easy exit at the end of service.

As the pastor was wrapping up the benediction, I turned to Mom and said, "It's time to go."

Mom looked at me and gave me a snappy, "No!"

I responded with, "Yes, Mom, we need to leave now."

Again, I got the no response. She then scooted to the right toward the other end of the pew. I scooted down as well, as she tried again. She scooted. I scooted. (Did I mention that the service was still taking place?) Fortunately, other worshippers had vacated the pew at this time.

By this time, we had scooted the length of the pew, and I had her wedged between me and the side of the pew, with nowhere else to go. Gently, I took her hand and asked her to come with me. Of course, she was pulling her hand out of mine. I was at my wits' end. Thankfully, the family sitting behind us intervened. They encouraged Mom to go with me and calmly guided her toward the end of the pew where we were first seated. An usher, watching from afar, had grabbed her wheelchair and positioned it in the aisle next to the pew. She got in, and we quickly rolled down the aisle and out of the sanctuary.

As we left the church, the helpful family simply said, "We'll be praying for you." I appreciated the sentiment but thought, *Would you like to take her for the day?* I thanked them for their help and their prayers. Angels are everywhere.

HER HEAVENLY GUARDIAN

For the most part, Mom had always been healthy and felt good most of the time. But bones grow brittle, accidents happen, and the bad days begin to outnumber the good.

Mom was living at her assisted living facility at the time of this particular accident. It is unclear what happened or when it happened, but sometime over the weekend, Mom fractured her sacrum. The sacrum is a large wedge-shaped vertebra at the lower end of the spine. It forms the solid base of the spinal column where it intersects with the hip bones to form the pelvis. The sacrum is a very strong bone that supports the weight of the upper body as it is spread across the pelvis and into the legs. Obviously, it is a significant bone. Once I found out she had been injured, I went on the warpath, but first, Mom had to go to the hospital.

I requested an ambulance to take her to the emergency room. Her pain was so intense that she needed morphine in order to be placed upon the gurney. She cried out in pain unlike I have ever heard before or since. I had never felt so helpless in my life. Mom always had a high tolerance for pain, but this time she was pushed beyond her capacity.

As we rode in the ambulance, I provided her health history to the paramedics and gave the approvals needed for treatment. I kept trying to comfort her and assure her that it would get better. The paramedics were very sympathetic and equally concerned about her comfort. They handled her as if she was a fine piece of crystal.

An x-ray was taken, which confirmed the fracture. Unfortunately, the only treatment for a fractured sacrum is time and pain management. The doctors said she would heal from it, but it would take a few weeks followed by physical therapy. They cautioned that giving her medicine for the pain could advance the dementia. Allowing her to suffer this way was not an option. We would deal with the disease later.

Her first night in the hospital was difficult. She would fall asleep for a few minutes and suddenly jerk awake because of the shooting pain in her lower back. Again and again, she would cry out and shake violently. For forty-eight hours straight I stayed by her side, gently holding her and silently praying until the pain subsided.

Even worse, Mom did not have the capacity to understand why she was hurting, just that she hurt.

Prayer is powerful. On the third day, I knelt beside my mother's bed and asked God to give me her pain—to not let her suffer this way. I asked him to give me her pain because I could take it and I would do anything to give her some relief. And in my prayers, I whispered to Mom that if this burden were too much to bear, I would let her go. I did not want her to leave me, but I would understand. I was her daughter and accepted the responsibility of taking care of her—no matter what. With tears streaming down my face, I finished praying and went to the restroom.

When I returned, her room was peaceful and serene. The whoosh and beeps of the medical equipment seemed to fade to simply background noise, instead of a constant reminder that someone was quite ill. As I approached her bedside, I gazed at the beautiful sight on her face: She was smiling at me! Her eyes were bright and clear. She seemed to recognize me and watched very carefully as I got closer to her. As I took her in my arms, my tears drenched her gown as I thanked God for intervening in our hour of need.

The next day, Mom was released from the hospital, and I was able to take her back to her assisted living facility. To this day, I'm still not exactly sure what the presence was in her room at that moment, but I know that God heard my prayers and blessed my mom and me once again.

REFLECTIONS

When I started caring for my mother in 1998, and eventually my father, I had little idea of what was in store. Frankly, I did not know what a caregiver was or how to prepare to be one. And I didn't think of myself as a caregiver—I was simply a loving daughter doing what she thought best for her parents.

I have since learned that women—including daughters, sisters, wives, and girlfriends—outnumber the men who serve in this role, which is understandable. After all, we are the nurturers and the ones called to keeping the family running smoothly.

After Daddy moved from the home he and my mother shared for so many years, he moved into the nursing floor, which was about four miles from the facility where Mom lived. Eventually, they made their way to the same facility but on different floors. A short time later, they made their way to living on the same floor and finally to sharing a room. Back together again. Somehow, we manage to have many family gatherings in that little space that rivaled anything we had when they lived in a five-bedroom house.

When Mom progressed to what is referred to as *end-stage dementia,* she lost her ability to walk or speak. She was unable to feed herself or tell me if she was uncomfortable. Yet people asked, "Cheryl, does she still recognize you?" At first, my first thought was, *Well that's a stupid question!* But I would simply smile and say, "Yes!" When I approached Mom, she stared at me for several seconds, then reached for my face and gave me the biggest smile possible. I know that somewhere, that vibrant, energetic, loving, and determined Miss Bee Bee was still in there. I honestly believe she knew me, but more importantly, I knew who *she* was. She was the woman who raised me, loved me, taught me right from wrong, and made me the woman I am today. She was loved and respected, regardless of whether she knew me or not. Of course, I missed our conversations, our adventures, our laughter, and our tears. But above all, I knew that I was privileged and grateful to care for her throughout her life.

A few years ago, a good friend asked me, "Are you prepared for how you will feel when God calls your parents home, after you have done everything possible to keep them comfortable, safe, and loved?"

My friend readily admits that he struggles to understand how I do all that I do, and still keep my head on straight. My answer? "No, I'm not prepared. I'm too busy living in the now to give that any thought. But when that happens, the greatest comfort for me as their daughter will be knowing that while they were on earth, I did everything within my power to advocate for the best care possible from the health care community."

I was devoted to making sure my parents had everything they needed to be comfortable and to thrive throughout this stage of their lives. This meant a triple-duty lifestyle—working full-time in a career that required travel, managing the operations of my home with my husband, and being supportive in the lives of my niece, nephew, and friends.

My sister, Lisa, and I made the sacrifices necessary to provide for them in a way that all of their basic needs were met. We celebrated birthdays, anniversaries, and all the big holidays. I picked up their laundry every three or four days and took it home, where I washed and ironed nearly every article of their clothing. Once completed, I delivered the fresh items back to them and put them away until next time. I estimate that I probably did about forty-five to fifty pieces of laundry each week for them alone. I made sure that their clothes and personal hygiene were always top-notch, for this is how they lived on their own. I visited them between four to six times a week, where we enjoyed each other's company and got caught up on the events of the day. It was my responsibility to get them to doctor's appointments, family gatherings, and any other events that occurred. Most evenings I did not arrive home until eight thirty. This may sound exhausting, but I was honored to provide this level of service to the two people I loved unconditionally.

I think about the times I challenged the doctors to provide them with full access to every single resource available in the medical community. I was a walking record of their medical histories, and I could quickly address any medical questions or concerns. And should a medical staff member determine care based on a quick assessment of their age or frequency of hospital stays—watch out! I was scarily calm as I expressed, in no uncertain terms and with great clarity and preciseness, exactly what I wanted for them, ending with my directive to extend, "every courtesy available that will support a full recovery." When it came to protecting my parents, I could teach a mama lion a few things about looking after her cubs.

I told my friend, "I was trying to do what my God commanded me to do. I always believed that whatever I needed to accomplish that, would be provided. I accepted the position with a devoted and humble spirit because I love them so! I cannot imagine anything else that gives me such pleasure and satisfaction."

My friend nodded in understanding and agreement as we both reached for a tissue and sat quietly for a few minutes.

BLESSED ASSURANCE

When I started recording stories about my relationship with Mom, I had no intention of putting them into a book. I merely wanted to preserve my precious memories. And truthfully, I was afraid that the end of my book would mean that my mother's life had come to an end as well.

On February 23, 2015, Mom made her final transition from this life and seventeen years of suffering from the debilitating effects of dementia. Throughout her lifetime, I witnessed the changes and challenges she faced as the disease took, bit by bit, her spirit, her energy, her cognition, and her love of life. For a woman who gave to others in numerous loving ways, it did not seem fair that her life would have come to this, but who says we are immune to sad or bad things? It is called life. There is a beginning and an end.

Dad and I were with Bee Bee when she made her departure from this life. For my entire life, I felt and believed that losing either one of my parents would be devastating for me. The mere thought of them dying would ignite an unbelievable pain, and I would not, could not survive it. I was wrong.

About a week before Mom's death, I spent time talking to her about her leaving us, assuring her that Lisa and I would continue to watch out for Daddy, and we all would be all right. I wanted her to stay with us—but not this way. I told her it was time for her to go to join Edna, Frank, Sue, Sam, Bob, and William. I stroked her head constantly and made sure she was comfortable, as I told her over and over how much I loved her and that she was an exceptional wife, mother, and friend.

During that entire week, there was not a moment where I felt fear or pain. I wanted my mom to be with me always, but only if she could live the life she had before her diagnosis. But that was not the plan God had for her. So I accepted His will, and at 12:03 a.m. on February 23, 2015, my promise to Miss Bee Bee was kept. She was at rest.

I called my husband, Larry, who was at home and told him that it was over. He had gone home hours earlier, but after getting my call, he immediately returned to be with Dad and me. We both waited for her tiny, sparrowlike body to be removed from her room by the funeral director. Dad, Larry, and I watched from a nearby window as Mom was rolled into the funeral transporter and driven out of sight.

My sister, Lisa, texted me a couple of hours later asking if Mom was still hanging on and I replied a simple no. She and Ralph were driving from Cleveland, hoping to get here before Mom's passing. I asked the funeral home to prepare Mom for Lisa's arrival so that she and Ralph could say their goodbyes as well.

Because we had done some prefuneral planning, the next steps were pretty simple. We laughed a lot about what Mom would and would *not* want. It was going to be a celebration of a life that touched many and who was loved by most.

We held a celebration of Mom's life on March 7, 2015, before a capacity audience that included family, friends, coworkers, and acquaintances. More than one hundred people came to pay their respects and share stories during the ninety-minute program.

There were many faces that Lisa and I did not recognize. Who were they, and what was their relationship with Miss Bee Bee? It was important to Lisa and me that those in attendance heard Miss Bee Bee's eighty-seven-year-long life story, not just the seventeen years of her diagnosis. With this goal as our foundation, my sister and I created a loving and tender tribute to our mother.

The professionals who took care of her during her ten years in Grand Rapids had one perspective. The life she had with our Dad for sixty-six years was full of energy, successes, insurmountable blessings, and yes, stories. Mom's nephews spoke about her as an aunt. My cousin Keith described her as fun and fearless, sharing a photograph of Mom attempting to ride a Big Wheel tricycle. Another cousin, Hans, talked about how God wanted her now to complete his bouquet and that from the moment she was born, he held February 23, 2015, just for her. We also invited Mom's supervisor from the Benton Harbor Housing Commission, Danethel Whitefield, to share stories of her professionalism, commitment, and generosity. Last, we asked Loraine Watson, Mom's closest friend, to speak about their relationship as best friends.

The service concluded with all the nieces, nephews, and in-laws singing a resounding refrain of "Blessed Assurance" led by my sister, Lisa. None of us are professional vocalists, and Lisa is not a trained choral director, but this never stopped us before. Soon the other guests joined in.

In the words of Paul Harvey, "Now, for the rest of the story." I had never told anyone that "Blessed Assurance" had a special meaning for Mom and me—one that eventually had me in giggles—because it was the song I would sing every time I had to toilet Mom. She would always claim that she did not "have to go," but once I got her on the toilet, I would start singing to her, "Blessed assurance, Jesus is mine ..." She would soon join in, and the water would flow. By the time the song was finished, so was her bladder. Others may have enjoyed our rendition of this time-tested hymn, but for me, it offered a visual in my head that is precious. If only my cousins could have seen the bubble above my head.

Three months after Mom's passing, I was out for an early morning spring walk. The trail is lined with magnificent fifty-year-old trees that create a dark, cavernous, tunnellike feel. The foliage is thick from years of continued natural growth. In the early mornings, a soothing silence engulfs the space. There is a particular place on this trail where

I feel one with my God, and I talk to Him about how grateful I am for all that He gives me to navigate this thing call elder care, and whenever I feel uncertain or afraid, I know He wraps me in blessed assurance.

The trail starts to curve toward the most magnificent clearing that opens into a wide space filled with a small pond, tall trees, and green spaces of tall grass and wildflowers. If I'm fortunate, I catch the sunbeams piercing through the trees. In this clearing, I talk to all the family members we have lost over the years. I call their names out loud: Grannie, Aunt Aretha, Joyce, Aunt Sue, and several more. I ask for their strength and guidance to help me make sure I am modeling the behavior they expect from me and tell them how much I miss having them in my life. But this time was different because I added Bee Bee's name to the list.

I openly sobbed for several minutes before regaining my composure. I cried because she was really gone, and my time with her was over. My 17-year journey, filled with stories and experiences, will replay in my memories of her for the rest of my life. Before she lost her ability to walk, we would take a leisurely stroll after dinner around a nearby lake. Mom marveled at the variety of colors along the way and pointed out things that I hadn't noticed. We had a favorite bench where we sat to watch the ducks and swans splash in and out of the water. After a few minutes, we continued with our walk. When she lost her ability to feed herself, I would step in to do that while I shared the events of my day. I wept for the years that she and my dad had to change their plans to travel and enjoy retirement together because of her illness. I wept because we were more than mother and daughter, she was my girlfriend.

I felt the warmth of the sun on my face, and it reminded me of the times, when Mom placed her hand on my cheek after she lost her ability to speak but could give me the most amazing smile. The smile that only a mother could give to remind how much parents love their children. As I moved through this pain of grief, I felt God's presence with me as well. Standing right beside Him was Miss Bee Bee—still four foot nine—telling me, "It'll be all right, baby."

So I have told my story about Mom, Miss Bee Bee. Now it is time to close this chapter by sharing how my life work has evolved. I believe that every life has purpose and a legacy to leave behind. No one is ever quite sure where our life paths will lead us, but if we don't follow them—or at least explore the journey—we may never know how each one can make an impact on others. Without a doubt, I believe that my life purpose is to be in service to others. Not too surprising since I seem to follow my mother's lead. I love interacting with seniors. Each occurrence allows me to share a bit of myself, but more importantly, I take a little part of them with me, which helps me to become a good steward for doing the work I am meant to do.

Therefore, I leave you with a summary of my "encore" season: *Where This Journey Has Led Me.*

I am gonna miss me some Miss Bee Bee. She was a good woman.

—Jerton Gray

WHERE THIS JOURNEY HAS LED ME

One summer day in 2013, my sister asked me when I was going to quit doing my eight-to-five job and start doing that one thing that I was intended for: a professional caregiver consultant. I looked at her with this look of disbelief and replied, "What do you mean?"

Lisa said, "You are never happier than when you are talking about caregiving and how you can plan and organize the challenges for others. You are not crazy about your job anyway, and frankly, they probably are not thrilled with you either. So quit!"

I said, "My household is dependent on two incomes, and the bank likes it when my husband and I make the mortgage payment each month."

Lisa simply said, "God will take care of that. Do not worry about it."

After the initial shock, I started to give it serious consideration and pondered the many possibilities that this could present for me. For the first time in my forty-plus-year career, I was contemplating launching my own organization designed around something that God had gifted me to do and that I thoroughly enjoyed.

Therefore, I enrolled in a program and earned a certificate in gerontology. Afterward, I created a business plan and talked to a number of sources to determine whether my idea had any merit. I received encouragement to keep moving.

The name of my company is Clear Path Choices, LLC. I have a team of people (collaborators, if you will) who assist me in creating care plans for families. Whether you are looking for placement or help with having that difficult conversation with a loved one, our mission is to help you navigate these challenges and survive. We provide the research and recommendations to ensure that you can make the best choice for your particular circumstance. Our clients receive a private and confidential consultation customized to each family's challenges.

The second piece we do is facilitate workshops for larger groups on the importance of planning life choices. *Decision Time* is a six-week seminar that helps individuals write down their decisions for their lives in one place for easy distribution to family, friends, and others who may be responsible for their care. Seminar participants learn from industry experts who provide accurate and up-to-date information. After the six weeks, all decisions are recorded in one place and can be easily updated as life changes occur. Simply put, "We help you find the way."

When I started my journey into (amateur) caregiving, little did I know what a whirlwind experience it would be. In the early years of this journey, I was very confused by the words and definitions of the health care community, the conflicting language of legal folks, and most of all the baffling vocabulary of the financial group. My head nearly spun off my shoulders trying to sort it all out.

However, my mother's well-being depended upon me to understand fully what all these different languages were saying to me. And eventually, I did—to great success. I did my research, networking, reading, and of course, praying. I created a library of resources that I could easily navigate and pull from for a whole variety of care solutions.

Soon I found myself developing expertise in being able to maneuver many of the obstacles people will face when it comes to taking care of someone who cannot take of him- or herself. About five years into this journey, I started coaching others and sharing what I had learned from my own experience. I effectively help them to create a path toward making important decisions for their and their loved ones' futures.

Because of the growing number of people entering retirement, resulting from the baby boomers hitting sixty years of age and older, the need for long-term care planning is critical. By the year 2030, there will be more people over the age of sixty living in this county than those younger than sixty, and society will undergo a significant change, as where we live, work, use disposable income, vote, and transport ourselves will shift dramatically. Taking the time now to plan for these changes in life choices will help to ensure that your needs will be met and that you can provide peace of mind to your family.

My parents understood the need for advanced planning. They sat me down and explained their legal, financial, and insurance conditions so I could make complete and informed decisions about their care. It is my desire to provide the same guidance and assurances to others. Making life decisions early on will help to reduce confusions, stresses, and conflicts. This makes way for enjoying the lives of those entrusted to your care.

RESOURCES

If you are looking for help to meet the demands of being a caregiver, these resources can help guide the way. Visit your local bookstore for additional information.

Memory Loss

- Mace, Nancy L., and Peter V. Rabins. *The 36-Hour Day: A Family Guide to Caring for People Who Have Alzheimer Disease, Related Dementias, and Memory Loss.* Baltimore, MD: Johns Hopkins University Press, 1999.
- Newmark, Amy, and Angela Timashenka Geiger. *Chicken Soup for the Soul: Living with Alzheimer's & Other Dementias: 101 Stories of Caregiving, Coping, and Compassion.* Cos Cob, CT: Chicken Soup for the Soul Publishing, LLC, 2014.
- The Alzheimer's Association. http://www.alz.org.

Caregiving

- Zukerman, Rachelle, PhD. *Alzheimer's for Dummies.* New Jersey: Wiley, 2003.
- Zukerman, Rachelle, PhD. *Eldercare for Dummies.* New York: Wiley, 2003.
- Morris, Virginia. *How to Care for Aging Parents.* New York: Workman Pub., 2004.
- Clear Path Choices: *We Help You Find the Way.* http://www.clearpathchoices.com/.

- AARP. www.aarp.org.
- The Family Caregiver Alliance. http://www.caregiver.org.
- Eldercare Locator. www.eldercare.gov.
- The National Alliance for Caregiving. www.caregiving.org.
- Rosalyn Carter Institute for Caregiving. rosalyncarter.org.

Elderly Care Resources
- Area Agencies on Aging (located in most counties across the country).
- Medicare. www.medicare.gov.

Printed in the United States
By Bookmasters